THE PRINCIPLES, ART AND PRACTICE OF HOMOEOPATHY

Dr. Trevor Smith

M.A., M.B.Chir., D.P.M., M.F. Hom.

INSIGHT

Insight Editions
WORTHING, Sussex
ISBN 0-946670-07-2

WARNING

The contents of this volume are for general interest only and
individual persons should always consult their medical
adviser about a particular problem or before stopping or
changing an existing treatment.

Printed and bound in Great Britain by
Biddles Ltd, Guildford and King's Lynn

THE PRINCIPLES, ART AND PRACTICE

OF

HOMOEOPATHY

"What Good is reason if it does not touch the heart?"

[King Arthur. Camelot]

CONTENTS

PART ONE

PART TWO

PART THREE

PART ONE

Chapter one

Introduction

Life is a blend of the infinitely changing, tangible and intangible, obvious and subtle, said and unsaid, definable and indefinable, hard and soft, love and hate, light and shade, similar and opposite, physical and mental. The one is more easy to talk about − the other less so. One is more amenable to words, communication, definitions, boundaries, understanding, saying than the other. Most of all, when we come to consider the psychological, it falls into the unsayable and the indefinable. Only its outer shell and external expressions − the *emotional*, enter more easily into the verbal, the outburst and the dramatic.

The doctor with his patient in the consulting room has to begin somewhere − with the facts of the case, the sayable, the words and hope that the softer, rounder, intuitive, deeper aspects of the 'case' will emerge given patience, goodwill, freedom from pressure, and co-operation. These 'other aspects', sometimes filtering through at the end, like the startling unexpected utterances at the door when a patient fills up to cry — only then, or after a pause full of meaning, also give in the closing seconds — the 'clue' to the remedy — "By the way doctor, I hope you don't mind me saying —". Sometimes a slip of the tongue or an odd peculiar symptom uniquely gives the remedy, just what is needed to confirm the prescription or sometimes to contradict and correct what was previously being formulated.

Beginnings are often rather factual, cautious, shy, clumsy, hesitant, predictable things and this is as true for the patient as for homoeopathy in general and for prescribing more specifically. Time is necessary to allow the deeper alternatives, the 'other' aspects, the new, the unique, to emerge into awareness and memory, for a communication based on trust and sharing — the doctor-patient relation-ship to develop. Once this has occurred then — and sometimes only then can the most appropriate remedy be formulated for the patient.

In the consulting room not too much attention should be given to the words alone. Body clues like movement and gesture must also be perceived as part of the overall communication. It is even a mistake to pay too much attention to the remedies that *at first* seem indicated. As the history proceeds and unravels — the physician needs to get an *overall* sense of what is happening, of what is said and left unsaid, for a balanced viewpoint and understanding of the within as much the without, so that a more subtle blend of facts and contact may occur with a depth and a *meaningful* contact. This can then stay, remain after the consultation and be an eventual brick to understanding and growth. This overall sense of totality is the homoeopathic aim of every caring consultation — which ultimately comes down to be a *meeting* in the fullest sense — a sharing of experiences, of contact, rapport between patient and doctor, of one human being with another.

For the patient, by the end of the consultation there should have been a clarification, understanding, something new, beyond the prescription, something indefinable. Call it insight, reassurance, 'interchange' but basically it is a sharing at some level, of one humanity with another, with a depth to it, and an interest. Looking at the outward shell of an internal problem and allowing for its existence — even when it cannot and be acknowledged, formulated or perceived, is part of the homoeopathic approach to every clinical problem however *apparently* superficial or trivial.

The aim of each communication is understanding, feed-back or response and the consultation is a communication which gives shape and form to an apparently meaningless clinical problem by individual advice and prescribing. The needs of patient and doctor are often not so different, distinct or even separable, — both ultimately seek understanding, knowing and truth.

The patient needs to know what homoeopathy is *really* about — its depths and boundaries and if it can help. The doctor needs to know the depths and boundaries of any internal blockages and pathological processes in order to prescribe. Both patient and physician alike need not just the lines of the illness but what is *between* them, what cannot always be said from lack of time or words or where levels and feelings are too painful, unsure, inprecise, philosophic or spiritual. But whatever the experience of the consultation, it is always necessary to complement words with feelings to give a depth and an intuitive sense, paving the way for a more solid realisations, experience and learning.

The *achievement* of such realisations is part of every homoeopathic consultation and should be an integral part of medicine in general — of *every* dialogue between doctor and patient, where the latter is more of a person, less of a child, the former more of a physician and friend, less a technician.

In this way consultations with the patient give potential for growth — one where blockages — physical or emotional can be sensed and discussed quite openly — the patient helped to see his own self-role, responsibility and contribution to his illness and problem, and that he is not just on the 'receiving end' of an attack by some *outside* invading force.

With greater sensitivity and awareness to what is happening beneath the surface, there can be more acceptance, more meaningful expression, contact and meeting in general as sensitivity is increased. In this way there is greater potential for change and growth, greater self-awareness and awareness of others, which is the ideal position for growth, development, maturity and health and an optimum psychological position for the remedies to act most advantageously.

Fullest self-realisation for the patient in the deepest sense is always the *ultimate* homoeopathic aim when considering cure.

Chapter two

The Principles of Homoeopathy

Without exception the highest aim of every sensitive physician must always be that which is best for his patient. This means not only resolution of physical problems but also an optimum psychological position of overall happiness and health. As far as possible the achievement of personal potential and abilities is desirable with a high degree of self-expression and expansion as an essential part of overall health and harmony.

Homoeopathy has always aimed for fullest personal development and self-realisation since its earliest days. It sees illness as the inevitable outcome of suppression and denial from a psychological viewpoint as well as physical stagnation, causing limitation and lack of wellbeing as the external manifestations of internal disharmony and diminished functioning.

Because of its infinitesimal dosage, individualisation of remedies that harmonise with
both psychological and physical aspects of the
patient, a doctor-patient relationship that
identifies with and recognizes the physical and
emotional needs of the patient, homoeopathy
can offer a truly biological alternative to the
increasingly synthetic mechanistic approach of
modern computerised medicine. It offers each
patient a safe, effective alternative to the many
potential dangers and side-effects of chemicals
increasingly used for every illness and which
are given more and more in isolation from the
patient as a person, who is seen increasingly as
a chemical disturbance only, with little account
taken of the human totality.

Illness is no easy matter for either doctor or
patient because of its many ramifications and
subtleties — past and present, organ as well as
cellular, physical as well as psychological. Each
level needs careful consideration before there
can be an understanding of the problem let
alone resolution of an illness and a return to
well-being.

No patient is a machine but a unique complex
evolving dynamic biological entity of varying
degrees of balance and harmony, externally
and internally. Particular consideration must
be given to the following factors whenever
vitality, balance, resistance or defence are undermined in order to come to a correct diagnosis
and eventually an effective remedy.

1. EXTERNAL FACTORS OF DISEASE

a) Physical

These include environment, climate, nutrition and diet, exposure to irritants or excesses of any kind which lessen or undermine essential functioning. The phases of the sun and moon may also be relevant to the onset or aggravation of certain conditions.

b) Other Organisms

These include all the normal inhabitants of man's environment with which in health he is in a balanced symbiotic relationship. These are the viral, bacteriological, plant, insect and parasitic worlds but also including the total micro- and sub micro-organisms which surround us constantly and usually interact in a smooth subtle way unless there is dis-harmony or dis-ease.

2. INTERNAL FACTORS OF DISEASE

a) Physiological

These include the rhythmic biological factors such as menstruation, the deeper-seated metabolic tides and rhythms and the acyclical factors like digestion, circulation, pulmonary functioning, urination, bowel-elimination and absorption.

b) Psychological

These include both the relationship to self as
well as to others. The inner world of conscious
and unconscious phantasy is constantly affecting us. It would destroy and dominate all
perception and understanding without the key
correcting role of the outer ego or perceptive
self which perceives the world of others and
reality much nearer to actuality than a
phantasy world would otherwise permit and
helps lessen blind certainty, black-and-white
assumption and absolute knowing.

c) Hereditary (see section page 28.)

d) Creative-inspirational

These deepest aspects of man are usually con-
ciously experienced as ideals, standards, faith
and morals or sometimes felt as what is most
God-like, excellent, caring and sensitive either
outside or within us. Where contact is lost with
these ultimate sources of being and there is loss
of faith, hope and belief then dis-ease may lead
to disease as vitality, resistance and drive to
live is lost.

Like the individual, homoeopathy is no easy
matter to understand, with complexities that
touch on and at times encompass the most
profound of man — his biological and physically unconscious as well as his psychological.
It encompasses an overall approach and view-

point of the individual and of that most evolved and complex form of living organisms and life — *homo sapiens* or man.

As modern man becomes increasingly mechanised, gadget-conscious, concerned with the outer and the immediate, the convenient and the short-cut, so less and less time, concern and acknowledgement is given to the slow the subtle, the intuitive and the unscientific or unprovable. Modern medicine has become increasingly identified with scientific progress, the measurable, the statistic, the electronic and the provable — the 'sterile' as much as the sterilised and increasingly remote from individual needs and contact.

Increasingly conventional medicine is blind to improvables and the intangibles of human contact, feelings and beliefs as well as fears. It is less a matter of healing and more one of nomenclature, pharmaceutical juggling and manipulation of physiological responses rather than aiming to support and enhance them in any way. The doctor-patient relationship is for the most part a thing of the textbook or theoretical workshop, as lack of time and group practice constantly crush to a minimum meaningful dialogue or ongoing contact, where insight, understanding, self-confrontation and realisation could occur or develop into *why* an illness has occurred and at this time.

In the last century Claude Bernard clearly defined individuality as a balanced ecological system with a vast continuous interchange of information and feed-back at every moment and at every conceivable level. Such multi-tiered information is also the major charac-teristic of the homoeopathic method and a full diagnosis can only be made by a synthesis of all the information available about reaction, coun-ter-reaction and internal balance. Especially in the emotional sphere, homoeopathy supports re-organisation, freeing and growth without stimulating any unnatural catharsis or dramatic temporary exit of feelings with no reference to the individual as a whole totality.

Violent, contrived and temporary exits of repressed emotional material or energy some-times occur in other therapies and are indeed their stated aim — imposing strains with little lasting therapeutic effect or value to the individual concerned. Homoeopathy with its minimal infinitesimal stimulus provides a more truly dynamising stimulus to re-organisation of the whole internal milieu in a natural way which harmonises with the real needs of the patient and his level of maturity. It acts in direct opposition to methods of the massive stimulus or the *mega* dose which only further diminish and suppress functioning, elimination and flow rather than giving essential support so that resolution and a return to balance can occur.

Homoeopathy is concerned with the global reactivation of the patient, putting into equilibrium all the biological systems by supporting and gently activating, stimulating functioning, flow, energy-movement and activity, whatever the need or depth. Where there is a mechanical blockage, then homoeopathy recommends a conventional or surgical approach rather than a stimulus to vital energy because the often dense nodal nature of such blockages, impoverished in vital energy within their centre makes them less responsive to homoeopathy. Usually homoeopathy plays a secondary supportive role until a mechanical constriction has been relieved.

Homoeopathy pays particular attention to the overall dynamic activity of each individual and to interference within this totality as part of its concern for the dynamic energy functioning needs of the patient. In this way homoeopathy assesses a remedy best suited for the patient's needs and for key support in a particular area when diagnosed as being deficient or where there is altered, lessened, diminished functioning and efficiency.

Psychological Factors in Illness

There is now general agreement that by far the most important trigger to *every* illness is the psychological one. Given sufficient time in the consultation it will emerge clearly enough but time, cooperation, a non-judgemental unpressurised attitude and patience are essential to clarify the picture. In the main, anxiety and emotional tension account for the common question which every patient asks "Why me — now?" As stress diminishes vitality, so too resistance is lowered with greatly increased susceptibility to external irritants even though benign, nevertheless lessening efficiency, functioning, flow and elimination.

Localised reactions of counter-irritation as heart-burn, flatulence, spasm, swelling, heat or redness are the body's attempts to redress balance. Not uncommonly there has been a similar exposure to fatigue, infection, cold or damp in a previous year, yet the patient remained quite well. At the time however he or she was not under pressure — with perhaps an interview or examination for promotion, a change of school, or a demand to perform and succeed with an added intolerable threat of failure, loss of prestige and love, so that failure was feared and seemed unthinkable. The parents may be also involved in a crisis, separated, divorced, re-marrying, creating further pressures and unknowns. Similarly a parent may be ill, senile or 'demanding' from a variety of reasons, all adding to the anxieties and giving extra stress to the sensitive child or adult.

It is not surprising that the intervention of a physical illness frequently saves face and self-image, putting off — perhaps once again, the agonising decision of 'What to do?' These are only a few of the many everyday factors that account for the timing of an illness. Anniversary reactions are when the timing, year, date of occurrence of a particular problem — either psychological or physical, have some significance or meaning to the original occurrence and trauma of earlier years.

Physical problems also of exhaustion, loss of interest, periods of debility may be the external expression of internal calendar events — the season, day, even hour relating to a stress or happening which was never fully come to terms with.

A 'problem' may have not been resolved in the past because it was denied at the time or because of traditional 'stiff upper lip' attitudes, that 'you don't show feelings', or 'not in front of the children' . In this way extremes of emotion may have been suppressed and denied, pushed under the surface only to re-emerge in later years as chronic recurrent problems that defy either diagnosis or cure. They have lost all obvious links to the original causes — their real meaning and purpose a hidden compromise-expression of the original trauma rather than an admission of pain, but at the cost of personal growth.

For others the possibility or even thought of a change of job or promotion poses a greater threat than redundancy. A new post is only seen as a pressure and exposure to possible failure. There is an overwhelming wish to change as well as to stay put and 'safe' — all of which causes anguish and fear. Refusing an offer may in reality be a 'last chance' — yet the risk of exposure, or a demand to perform are quite dreaded, and have been throughout life.

Openness, spontaneity, sharing, on-going discussions in the present — cannot be over-emphasised as major factors in preventing any build-up of nervous tension. The perspectives given aid considerably in the resolution of a denied or delayed problem which would otherwise become a nagging source of worry, stress and uncertainty. There is much truth in the old adage of 'a worry shared is one halved'. Discussion of every unknown, new and unfamiliar situation is an enormous boon to confidence and helps prevent phantasy from excessively dominating reality view-points.

For every individual, without exception, getting things into perspective is essential for health and avoids a new unfamiliar experience becoming one of alarm and panic. Lack of discussion and dialogue are the most common reasons for inappropriate excessive reactions where stress and pressure become danger and fear.

Physical Factors in Illness

Pressure and exposure to outside physical stimulus can cause disastrous internal injury or damage to tissues when in excess. All the elements, given conditions of massive exposure, reduce vitality and increase susceptibility. They can precipitate a localised cellular reaction, even one of deep organ involvement where the body fails to contain the irritation and damage at local levels. Lumbago if severe, may move deeply into the kidneys; tonsillitus may gain the lungs; a common cold move deeper into the sinuses from the nose or throat. Exposure to excessive dryness or heat can be just as dangerous as cold and damp and equally damaging.

Vulnerable organs like the heart or lungs can sometimes be permanently damaged when the patient is caught 'off guard', not properly protected or in a vulnerable depleted condition and then even mild exposure can lead to permanent weakness. Trauma of any kind, from a bruise or local pressure can not only damage tissue but in a weakened state be the trigger to more generalised reactions of shock and collapse. This then becomes an added complication to the existing clinical picture and a further problem for the patient.

When such shock reactions are severe as in acute fear, their effects may be far more important, far-reaching and lasting than those of the actual physical damage.

Case Report:

A patient seen recently after a cataract operation developed a swelling of the face and eyelids on the opposite side of the face to the operation. She realised in the consultation that psychologically she had experienced the surgery as a personal assault and that in spite of the improved vision had become quite ill. There had once before been a similar minor surgical procedure, also associated with the same feelings of personal damage. when she had reacted with a post-operative urticarial illness. In this case the remedy needed was *Staphisagria* because of the high degree of resentment as well as tissue disturbance and it quickly led to rapid improvement of all symptoms.

But in other cases the psychological outcome of such trauma only occurs weeks or months after the event. It is always essential to get the origins and associations as clear as possible, to avoid chronic problems from developing and to resolve the roots of any associated emotional feelings. The homoeopathic remedy helps bring such reactions to the surface and can then free them sufficiently to allow their expression and clarification in this way facilitating resolution and cure. Suppressed symptoms and reactions of this type are often totally repressed or forgotten — sometimes not experienced again for many years. Physical or psychological in type, it is only as the remedy rolls back the underlying layers and brings them up to the surface that they are consciously recalled and can be permanently dealt with. The unearthing of such reactions is of particular importance in the treatment of many undermining, chronic states which lower resistance and vitality until released in their true perspective by the correct homoeopathic potency.

Hereditary Factors in Illness

Inherited areas of susceptibility, weakness and vulnerability are the Achilles heel of every patient. Especially where there is a chronic disease problem genetic make-up may sap quite specific areas of functioning and pathways of energy producing a variety of symptoms sometimes in other members of a family with lack of energy, vitality and weakness. Such susceptibility may clearly run through several generations and lead to greatly increased sensitivity to a variety of substances otherwise perfectly harmless. These external triggers include house-dust, insect stings or specific flower pollens and may evoke severe, sometimes dangerous allergic reactions. In others it is hyper-sensitivity to a synthetic substance that is inherited, with inability to reduce and excrete otherwise benign factors from lack of an essential factor in the intracellular enzyme chain which breaks down complex substances into simpler ones for excretion. Colorants, preservatives, pesticides, herbicides, oxidisers, tenderisers, pharmaceutical synthetics are only some of the chemicals that may accumulate in this way and build up to critical levels so that eventually the slightest amount provokes a severe chain-reaction and physiological crisis.

Migraine from 'sensitivity' to food-factors like chocolate, cheese or gluten can also act in a similar way at intracellular levels from an enzymic failure to convert them to more simple compounds for excretion.

The psychologist Adler described such familiar inherited factors as 'organ weakness'. Others have called them familial, hereditary predispositions or constitutional weakness. Certainly constitution and inheritance are closely linked. The homoeopathic theory of hereditary miasms describes a constitutional flaw carried by a genetic carrier factor from one generation to another and expressed as well-recognizable patterns of chronic diminished functioning. The weakness, with lows of energy and symptoms bears a superficial but clear resemblance to the original suppressed illness but without either its epidemic morbidity or contagious characteristics.

Such miasmic constitutions are best treated by the appropriate homoeopathic remedy in high dilution. Psora is the major group and increasingly in every age group its contemporary expression as psoriasis has become a therapeutic challenge to every doctor. Similarly familiar predisposition to asthma, eczema, hayfever and allergy in general are other common external manifestations of deep-seated internal problems with an underlying miasmic thread to account for their chronicity. Failure to respond to a variety of treatments is usually because these fail essentially to get to grips with the underlying depths and real causes of the illness.

Congenital Factors in Illness

Congenital factors are closely related to hereditary ones and are areas of malformation or incomplete development from viral causes like rubella and other unknowns during the inter-uterine phase of growth and development. The problems include cystic formation within the kidneys, patent or unclosed channels or walls within the circulation or heart structure or only partial developments in less vital areas as the genitals. The patient is born with these deficiencies or limiting factors to a varying degree and in general corrective surgery is the only approach at as early a stage as possible. Where they have not been diagnosed until late in life such abnormalities of growth can often be responsible for a wide variety of chronic problems and puzzling symptoms. Treatment is either conservative with homoeopathy playing a major role, or corrective surgery with homoeopathy in a background supporting position.

Chapter three

Symptoms and the Patient

Symptoms are the diagnostic bricks of homoeopathic practise and the essentially healthy dynamic response to internal inbalance by the patient. The practitioner builds up diagnostic profiles from these overall symptom patterns which give the picture of individual dynamics. These can then be compared with the 'proving' or toxicity profiles of various remedies which are the typical physiological reactions to the remedy in its unprepared and undiluted natural form. The best 'match' most completely resembling the symptoms is chosen as the prescribed medicine.

A symptom is what patients feel and experience about themselves. It is what tells them that all is not right and that they may need help or advice. The most common symptoms initially are often the most vague — a sense of tiredness, diminished general interest, sexuality and functioning, lack of efficiency or concentration, malaise, irritability and frequently inability to relax during the day or to sleep at night. In some cases overactivity takes the place of the

29

more typical lethargy and an upsurge of energy makes relaxation or sleep impossible. These are the *general* — or early non-specific symptoms of the individual involving the whole of the body system and common to every illness in some way or other but not a useful basis to prescribe upon or to make a diagnosis.

The *specifics* are much more definitely related to an organ or part of the body — as pain in the great toe of an acute gouty condition, or pain in a knee or joint with swelling, perhaps immobility, in a rheumatoid condition.

Other *specifics* might be swelling of a facial salivary gland in mumps or a definite distinctive rash in measles. Some symptoms are not so easily defined or definitely related to any known previous condition, joint or organ — even to a part of the body, yet they feel real and tangible enough. Examples of these odd and peculiar symptoms are a sense that the body is made of glass or has a live animal inside it. (*Thuja*) In others the whole of the pelvic organs seem to be dropping and the legs must be kept tightly closed to prevent this happening. (*Sepia*) Such odd symptom-specifics have a maximum value in prescribing and are especially highly valued by the diagnosing homoeopathic physician.

Because these very early symptoms are so vague and uncertain, easily overlooked with only a general sense of feeling fatigued, exhausted, below par, jaded and irritable, a specific diagnosis is not always possible either in terms of pathology and cause or any indicated remedy because the body at this stage has not yet fully mobilised its own defensive reactions which produce the more clear-cut diagnostic symptoms. The classical clinical picture is not present to confirm or otherwise a pathological condition and its treatment.

At this early stage specific illness is usually also absent — in terms of organ disfunction and therefore laboratory confirmation of diagnosis is often absent too. It is here that homoeopathy scores above all other treatment methods because the prescription can be effectively initiated well before major changes occur in key organs and cellular centres. The homoeopathic approach completely supports such early reactions well before later more massive changes have occurred at macroscopic level, in this way preserving, protecting and supporting essential organs, cellular entity and functioning to a maximum.

In order to understand a diagnostic problem, a maximum of time is essential for the consultation, especially during these early 'incubating' phases where the body is *just* out of phase and balance because energy flows and vitality are deviated to pressure areas without the tangible appearance of any diagnosable clinical condition. This can be a worrying phase for doctor and patient alike. Both know that 'something' is wrong but neither is quite sure just what the problem is. It is for such problems

— intangible and uncertain that the homoeopath uses the 'high' intangible potencies of 200c and more to either support and rectify or otherwise clarify the underlying situation.

Symptoms may occur which only others perceive rather than the patient himself. They see a change in basic personality, perhaps of reasoning or logic, a preoccupation with certain themes or mannerisms, changes in patterns of sleep or temperament, a tendency to withdraw and solitude beyond the expected or usual norm for the individual concerned, their past habits and patterns.

The doctor may be consulted about such changes by relatives rather then the patient who fails to perceive them as symptoms needing help or any possible illness or toxic state. This may quite commonly occur in an acute psychotic disorder from toxic, infective, febrile or puerperal causes. An acute traumatic condition or pressure build-up situation may also be a cause in vulnerable sensitive temperaments. A sudden degenerative state may similarly affect perception and reality-interpretation with distortion of all outside sensations and experiences. In this way the patient comes to live in a delusional world of phantasy and unreality, without realising it.

There may be over-concern with appearance, body size or boundaries of self. Imaginative phantasy-ideas dominate to such an extent that there is neglect of basic body needs of nutrition and hygiene and the increasing isolation becomes a source of worry to the family. There are no generalised recipes or rules for such problems and each must be assessed and dealt with on its merits, as throughout homoeopathy the individual comes before all other considerations.

Whatever the problem or its manifestation, the patient remains primarily a person, an individual and this must be respected and treated accordingly. Only rarely, when the patient is a danger — to themselves or others, refusing all help and treatment-endeavours or opposing them, should a legally compulsory consultation and treatment be imposed. Such measures run the risk of aggravating the condition and are best reserved for the most desperate uncontrollable situations. When needed, homoeopathy nevertheless stands by its principles of respecting the needs and individuality of the patient, prescribing on the totality rather than on any pathological name or psychological syndrome. Where the problem is unmanageable and acute, homoeopathy may have to be combined with sedation or kept in reserve until a violent phase has lessened its intensity.

Every symptom — no matter how extreme, urgent or bizarre is the healthy reaction of the body to distress and pressure of some kind which threaten internal harmony. It is always the body's attempt to redress the balance and a move towards healing. Symptoms imply a healthy vital response, one to re-create physiological or psychological normality and homoeostasis.

The absence of symptom-reactions is always a matter of grave concern and may reflect an absence of energy reserves as can occur in certain toxic exhaustive states where vital energy and response is minimal. This is quite common in the elderly but equally may be seen in a child where there is overwhelming weakness as when vulnerable and convalescent, or an infection has very great force and toxicity as in some forms of epidemic pneumonia or meningitis. In these cases the temperature may be sub-normal, the patient collapsed or shocked without vital response and weakening hour by hour.

A similar serious situation can also occur when a massive infection occurs in the wake of a debilitating condition as after hepatitis, glandular fever or whooping cough with the patient in a vulnerable weakened state. Infections like typhoid, cholera, chicken pox or measles can be much more severe in the adult or where general resistance is low, reserves and energy minimal so that there is little defence against overwhelming toxicity.

According to homoeopathic theory, whatever the illness or manifestation, the mind first and foremost is in disarray creating the ideal conditions for the externals like infection, invasion, inflammation, weakness, to gain access or take root. The very deepest aspects of man — the creative-inspirational cannot be blocked, only its outlets of expressions may be deviated. Especially, symptoms like vagueness, loss of energy, irritability, depression or anxiety may be the outcome of such deviation or sometimes lead on to loss of personal faith, conviction, creative drive or interest. Associated flattening of all that is 'highest and best' occurs so that the inspirational as well as psychological satisfactions are minimal. The alternative pathways available are inevitably less satisfying because they provide indirect and only limited partial outlets to creativity and psychological expression often adding to existing uncertainty, tension and frustration rather than relieving them.

Chapter four

Some General Points Concerning Symptoms and Prescribing

In every case have a scheme of approach and history-taking but keep it flexible — a framework only, not a rigid package, recording major symptoms in the patient's own words. Always be prepared to change a formulation as the history develops and becomes clearer. Repertorise when in doubt and use the remedy which occurs most frequently and consistently, but always leave the final decision of *which* remedy to the end of the consultation. Where the repertorised remedy and your own intuitive remedy are not the same, be prepared to act on judgement and experience rather than any reference manual, however, good, especially where there is doubt.

Always consider the possibility of an organic non-homoeopathic condition where symptoms are not the response and outcome of stasis and stagnation of vital energy and where the whole physiological system seems to be in revolt or straining desperately to overcome blockage — pouring out mucous, fluid, blood, through every pathway and physiological circuit available to it.

In cases of 'organic' tissue changes or blockage — as from scar-tissue, stroke or embolus, only prescribe homoeopathically where conventional treatment is not better indicated or has failed. For such conditions consider 'local' treatment with remedies in 'low' potency providing they fit the overall picture. Always be alert to a possible organic condition needing conventional treatment — medical or surgery as the action of choice for the patient rather than homoeopathy.

When in doubt, be prepared to refer to an orthodox colleague or where homoeopathy is not working or should perhaps be in a more supporting role rather than the prima donna. Insistence on any one method for such cases and omnipotence by the physician is neither homoeopathic, holistic, or therapeutic and goes agains homoeopathic principles where the interests of the patient always come first and not the method.

A More Detailed Evaluation Of Symptoms For Prescribing

1 Never prescribe for either an acute or chronic physical condition without first considering the mentals and confirming the remedy by making quite sure that there is accurate 'fit' of the prescription in this area as much as in the physical one.

2 Never prescribe for either an acute or chronic psychological condition without considering any associated physical symptoms and making certain that the remedy 'fits' in this area as much as in the mentals.

3 When symptoms are 'mixed', the history both acute as well as chronic, prescribe for one set of symptoms only, according to clinical judgement — usually those most severe and acute.

4 Never prescribe on the side-effects of a synthetic remedy as if representing a true expression of the body's vital reaction — like extreme sleepy fatigue from anti-histamines. Regard these as artefacts and not true prescribable dynamic reactions of the patient giving any accurate indication for the remedy.

5 At all times only prescribe for the individual's vital reaction. Prescribe a synthetic remedy in potency — eg *Librium* 30 or *Valium* 30 where symptoms date back

to first taking these — and the patient never well since that time.

6 Don't come to a definite decision as to the best remedy for the individual until you have heard *all* the complaints and the consultation has ended — allowing time in the final minutes for significant new material to come in at the end and if necessary to influence the choice of remedy. Note any major remedies, as the history unfolds in the margin of the case notes but leave the final choice as late as possible in the consultation time. If necessary only decide later and repertorise where there is doubt.

7 If the patient gives a physical or otherwise diagnostic label at the beginning of the consultation, don't be influenced by it in terms of the homoeopathic prescription. Explain to the patient that each remedy is based on quite specific patterns of vital reaction and symptoms — not on diagnostic labels and terminology.

8 In every case, try to go back to the earliest origins of both illness and patient whenever possible. Where this is difficult — perhaps with an early infantile eczema of obscure origin, always look for familial miasmic factors or known external precipitating triggers like animal hair, pollen or house-dust.

9 Pay particular attention to psychological factors especially in the more chronic serious problems as diabetes, cancer, colitis, peptic ulceration, degenerative conditions, heart attack or angina pectoris, letting these emerge gently and spontaneously, as the case develops, trying with the patient to understand the importance, significance, meaning, roots and associations of the illness.

10 Where the clinical picture is not clear enough to prescribe for by the end of the consultation, especially with a long history of multiple allopathic suppressant treatments or too frequent doses of homoeopathic potencies, it is often useful to give placebo for a time provided that it is in the best interests and needs of the patient. A second consultation should then be arranged without undue delay to further clarify the symptoms and history. Others need a remedy like *Sulphur* to clear the terrain and provoke a vital reaction to clarify the present position so that more accurate specific individual prescribing can be commenced as early as possible.

Chapter five

The Mentals and Homoeopathy

'Understanding the mind of the patient is key to understanding the man and the roots of his illness' — emphasised Hahnemann 200 years ago, giving fundamental importance to psychology in his approach to the individual – a century before Freud. From the start homoeopathy paid detailed attention to mental attitudes, especially the most limiting ones like fear, anxiety, guilt and obsessional control. The total psychological aspects of the person are grouped in homoeopathy as the *mentals* and include habitual attitudes to both self and others; patterns of relationships as well as defences against them; perception of self and others; controls — either excessive or absent and lacking whatever the provocation or situation. Every patient needs particular attention to be given to all these areas especially where there are rigid attitudes which limit or reduce spontaneity, essential closeness, expression and contact. When these are severe and not allowed to emerge, they can become barriers to cure and resolution of a problem area or act as triggers to the onset of illness. They may undermine any homoeopathic effect provoking sudden exacerbation or crisis with severe physical symptoms from no outer obvious cause or provocation. In such cases, where inner mental attitudes are obscure or undeclared, this adds to the difficulty of the physician to handle and treat the exacerbation until the underlying psychological mental has been unearthed.

Case History 1

A patient seen recently with severe chronic facial and body eczema showed a marked improvement with high potency *Pulsatilla*. Week after week the condition lessened and after two months she was 90% better. She was living with a rather dominant over-anxious husband however who 'swallowed her up' psychologically speaking. She was never seen alone or without his presence and fears. There was a lot of underlying resentment at this state of psychological affairs and although the skin level of the problem cleared quickly with homoeopathy the internal mental dynamics had not shifted significantly. Suddenly and without any obvious reason or provocation the whole eczema condition flared-up again, but much more severely this time than ever before, associated with 'swallowed' feelings of internal resentment. The previous improvement lacked the depth to contain and modify the eczema, although clinically the skin condition had seemed outwardly better.

Case History 2

A patient came with a two-year history of attacks of violence and loss of control, improving markedly with *Nux Vomica*. The attacks of the past were quite clearly related to hypoglycaemia caused by delayed luncheons or working late at the office without food. On one occasion he accidently banged his head on a cupboard and became enraged, smashing-up the cupboard in fury. Later that same afternoon he became involved in a violent argument with another motorist who followed him home when he had earlier suddenly pulled out in front of him.

Following an outburst of shouts and threats my patient became completely exhausted as well as agitated for two weeks or more before again calming down. In this case again, the overwhelming strength of underlying attitudes and poor controls had not been sufficiently 'held' by the remedy – although in high potency and accurate. The psychological problems still needed much more time to consolidate, emerge and strengthen before there could be outer changes in behaviour and control.

The 'trigger' to a breakdown of rigid controls is often alcohol, fatigue, low blood sugar or synthetic drugs which upset the whole system. Deep acting allopathic remedies like sedatives, tranquillisers, anti-histamines may relieve symptoms but they also undermine well-being and are addictive in a way that homoeopathy never is. Such synthetics commonly provoke as side-effects the very problems that they seek to relieve, creating added confusion as well as anxiety and dependence for the patient to additionally cope with.

Visions, ideas of reference and feelings that others are influencing and acting upon them in some way is always a matter of concern for the physician. Also hallucinations, delusions, states of 'clairvoyance', paranoid feelings, or conviction beyond doubt − despite reality and fact must all be assessed as part of an overall totality. It is always important to decide whether a psychotic state has developed or not and any break with reality. The degree, intensity, preoccupation, withdrawal and patterns of relationships, contact, expressions as well as spontaneity all give the clue to the severity of a particular set of symptoms and how serious the disturbance of personality and its depth.

The cooperation of the patient, degree of humour and insight are also important in deciding just what dominates the mind and whether the primitive internal phantasy-world has completely broken through and taken over. Outward emotional strain and tension may only be a temporary and relatively superficial indication of prevailing stress-pressures which the individual is trying to suppress and control as well as resolve in his or her unique way. The less tangibles like mistrust or jealousy, are also important areas for consideration, to understand and clarify where they distort or undermine essential trust and contact — best seen as part of the overall general approach to the whole person and not taken too much in isolation.

Any change of temperament in recent months especially following a history of infection, head-injury, concussion, epilepsy, 'black-outs' or 'fits', or where a dissociated state of 'absence', incontinence, or of temporary weakness and loss of control has occured, needs careful assessment. A proper balanced appraisal, accurate diagnosis, prescription or referral must always be made. If a pattern has changed without obvious cause or provocation in a person of previous stable make-up, then this must be taken as a cause for concern and taken seriously to exclude the possibility of a cerebral new growth, primary or secondary from another area of the body as the lung, breast or prostate — possible infective or neoplastic. In such cases a full and early investigation may be required with body or brain scans for early diagnosis and treatment.

When there is doubt, the needs of the patient take priority over all other considerations and without hesitation a surgical or neurological opinion should be sought at an early date. It may be a mistake in such cases to prescribe homoeopathically in 'high' potency until organic causes have been either eliminated or clearly diagnosed — to avoid loss of valuable time in a possible surgical condition or an aggravation which has no therapeutic value to the patient because of an obstructive condition. Where homoeopathic help has been sought far too late in the evolution of an illness for a curative response to be possible, it is also a mistake to prescribe 'high' or to attempt other than secondary supportive measures because a healing vital reaction is unlikely or impossible.

Any changes in long-established physiological patterns or rhythms — of bowel or digestive organs — where it has never previously occurred and there is no obvious cause, must always be thought about deeply, and organic underlying 'hidden' pathology excluded as soon as possible. Mechanical conditions of an organic type are not usually so amenable to the homoeopathic method and are usually best dealt with by other conventional methods. Because such problems may so closely mimic a psychological disturbance, their exclusion from the mentals is always in the patient's best interests as well as for homoeopathic prescribing.

Dreams are the symbolic language of the unconscious mentals and give conscious expression to them in an attempt to contain and resolve physical as well as psychological blocks in a pictorial symbolic way. They encompass a great deal of the patient's present preoccupations and mental happenings as well as deeper, unconscious, 'forgotten' or unknown motivations and drives. The dream compresses within it both the recent trigger or provocation as well as the remoter root-causes and origins from the past. Dreams have a further purpose beyond the simple repetition of a theme however because they attempt resolution of the problem by a symbolic compromise which preserves both sleep as well as peace of mind. In many cases the compromise has no value at a realistic conscious level although for some there is the added bonus of actual problem-solving by the dream of an acute difficulty as well as being an ally to equanimity.

In every dream it is important to know whether the dreamer is participating in the dream-theme and activity or if remaining an onlooker. This gives a clue to the degree of involvement in general of the patient with their underlying mentals as well as the amount of denial and suppression. Where passivity is marked, the patient a total observer − then this may indicate a minimum of active participation with unconscious themes and an attempt to distance themselves from everyone because they are felt to be overwhelming.

The symbolic meaning of the dream gives an important clue to the underlying mentals as well as to relationships in general and may indicate a specific remedy. Every level of information given by the patient should be constantly assessed without applying either formula or recipe and seen as a potential clue to the remedy as well as a positive attempt by the patient to regain equilibrium, resolution and balance. Especially note any nightmares or waking-dreams and those that repeatedly express a theme or particularly vulnerable 'dangerous' position.

Some Examples Of Dreams And Their Associated Remedies

Dreams of dogs and general anxiety-fear situations — *Belladonna*

Dreams about business problems and worries — *Bryonia*

Severe anxiety dreams — *Arsenicum, Lachesis*

Dreams of ghosts — *Sulphur, Carbo veg, Pulsatilla*

Dreams of the dead or dying — *Kali carb, Thuja*

Where there are more specific sleep disturbances — see what form they take and whether there is waking at a particular time and how this relates to a particular remedy under consideration, as well as to overall physical symptoms and make-up – either confirming a particular remedy or otherwise.

Examples Of Remedies With Their Specific Pattern Of Insomnia

Arsenicum — waking at midnight or from 12.— 1.00 am

Pulsatilla — waking between 2 – 3.00 am - often feeling too warm and hungry

Nux vom — waking at 3.00 am

Kali carb — waking at 4 – 5.00 am

Lycopodium — unable to get off to sleep because of an over-active mind usually pre-occupied with anticipated future problems.

In every person, always assess the direction and form that the underlying mentals are taking. For example moving more deeply from an obsessional-compulsive problem into a delusional–paranoid state, or more superficially from an obsessional-phobic position to one of increased anxiety but also greater mobility, relaxation and superficial fear. The underlying intensity of the feelings expressed should always be explored and known about as well as acknowledged, by the patient. In this way deep-seated or denied emotion and stress can be helped from going deeper or taking a more serious turn, where it is more difficult to treat because it is less accessible, remote from discussion, dialogue and remedy action.

If there is any tendency for this to happen with increasing depth and frequency of symptoms or withdrawal then the remedy, provided that it still 'fits' the major symptoms, should be increased substantially in potency to a higher 200 C or a 10 M to be able to reach these deepening tendencies. If the remedy no longer 'fits' then another should be re-prescribed in the higher potency as indicated above. Where the move is to more positive available levels of expression, with substantial lessening of unreality, delusion and conviction, then the remedy should be continued unchanged and not interfered with or re-prescribed as long as the patient is improving.

With every patient, whatever the problem, try to gain maximum insight into the mentals, their direction and outward form as well as any internal phantasy-preoccupations which may limit expression, development and functioning. The moves may at times be into a 'high' phase of excitement or an exalted one of optimism and energy. In others it can equally be the reverse and a 'down' phase of depression, lethargy and withdrawal.

In every case without exception the aim of the homoeopathic physician is the fullest possible realisation of the individual, his or her potential and gifts — expressive as well as creative, whatever their form, uniqueness and metaphor.

Chapter six

On the Causation of Mental Illness

Modern man is largely alienated from his true self – aims, beliefs, directions and depths, as much ill at ease with himself as with others.

Man panics as much at the inevitable outer social changes as the more inner psychological ones. Like his macrocosm, society, he is rarely flexible enough when faced with the new or prepared for it. Rigid up-bringing as well as inflexible educational methods perpetuate the early omnipotent beliefs that life, relationships, industry and man himself are both fixed and unalterable. Because of these reassuring assumptions man is never prepared for the changes that inevitable occur, is suprised by them when they come and most of the time is caught 'off-balance'.

It is wrongly assumed that all life is an extension of the past — both a direct continuation and dependent upon it rather than an *emerging* journey into the new and the changing — the developmental and the unfolding. Education teaches us the rule of the definite and the dogmatic, the theorem and the maxim, denying at the same time the constant exceptions that occur at every turning of the way and with every new experience. When change comes man is shaken and unprepared, does not know how to approach it and too quickly gets into a panic state. He takes flight into neurotic patterns of self-destruction and repetition with little that is positive to support the new attitudes required to understand, harmonise and respond. Neurotic weakness patterns attempt to deny the new, the changing, the reality. It is directly opposed to growth from experiences as they occur — gaining strength and knowledge through them so that a *real* maturity can emerge out of problem solving and confrontation with lessening of infantile omnipotence and fear, the root of every emotional illness and neurosis.

Chapter seven

On the Positive Value of Symptoms

Pain

Every acute condition, by mobilising vital energy into the area — for example a scald, burn, boil or abscess, serves an important balancing and defensive function and naturally supports positive reactions of protection and withdrawal in a damaged area which otherwise might be ignored or neglected. Where a degenerative condition exists, or an accident has caused severence of pain-conducting pathways, even a mild burn or scald can become quite a severe crisis. Where pain is absent – it may become either neglected or knocked, quickly infected and ulcerated or a burn occur on the same or neighbouring site increasing the original depth and damage. This occurs in some cases of multiple sclerosis where a burn causes no experience or sensation of pain because there is damage to spinal temperature pathways and repeated tissue damage is a risk because of diminished sensation as a warning sign. Although pain is generally considered a negative and disagreeable thing, in fact it has a very important positive protective function and its absence can be much more of a problem that its presence.

Redness

Local signs like burning heat and redness in the area warn the patient of the extent of a problem, its localization, advance or decline and delineate the extent of damage. It also acts like an early-warning sign, supporting the need for care, attention and rest, in this way supporting healing.

Swelling

Fluid accumulation in local tissues causes swelling and pain as the encapsulating tissues and nerves of the area affected are stretched to their limit and under pressure. There is however a protective cushioning effect as the fluid infiltrates into the area. Another factor is immobilisation from the fluid which helps avoid sudden damaging movements because of stiffness and pain − in this way also supportive. Internally increased fluids provide an important pathway for the body's fighting troops − the white cells or leucocytes. As well as a point of entry for them by the increase in circulation it also gives a key exit for dead material − toxic or dead cells which must be removed to avoid infection or chronic irritation accumulating. Later the scavenger lymphocytes clean up the area also using the same pathway of entry and removal. Swelling tells the patient what is happening in the area — where and how long a condition is lasting. In this way it has an important function for health.

Discharges

Although often thought of as repugnant, unpleasant things they too play a major role in drainage and general cleaning-up of an area of infection or damage. They provide vital information as to the advance or decline of an infected area as well as the progress of vital energy and healing reactions. The colour, consistency, odour, amount and frequency tells both patient and doctor about the acuteness or otherwise of a condition in addition to its action as an important exit for potentially damaging toxic material.

Chapter eight

Taking the History

With every patient a full history must be taken of the details of the case and records kept of progress or otherwise. In homoeopathy the history is even more detailed and extensive than usual because of attention given to detailed symptoms and the evolution in depth of the illness in order to reach a correct diagnosis and prescription. There should be a full description in the patient's own words of the tangible symptoms, their onset, site, patterns and modalities — as well as of any factors which either alleviate or aggravate the condition. The intangibles must be recorded as clearly as possible — their pattern, frequency and any relevance to the illness because of their often major importance in early diagnosis of either an organic condition or a psychological one. Both may need to be carefully and clearly differentiated at an early stage. Anything the patient has noted, has on their mind or cannot perhaps understand or relate to, is important and may be significant however seemingly minute or trivial at the time. Some remedies have such odd-peculiar symptoms as part of their make-up and when these come into the history and the rest of the symptoms 'fit', it is highly likely that this particular remedy is the one indicated for the patient — either immediately or at some time in the future.

In history taking, what matters is to try to understand the patient as an individual — a person and not just as a collection of symptoms or an illness. Try to get an overall meaning of the totality of what is said and described, the meaning of an illness within the individual life-pattern as well as life-style. Note any fears that the illness evokes, why and how these are coped with. Attitudes of optimism, humour – positive as well negative should be recorded as they may give an important clue to psychological health. It always matters when the patient was last fully well and any relevant earlier factors, like vaccination, head-injury, shock or a physical illness as glandular fever, mumps or influenza that occurred. Drugs taken at the time of onset and since may have affected overall balance and health when there is allergy or sensitivity and the patient never fully recovered or well since.

Aim to see every illness in terms of overall development, aspirations, goals, expression and attainment as well as any blockage or interference that may have occurred. Look at each problem both physically as well as psychologically and see the inner man whenever possible, discussing this with the patient in an *open* way so that he or she can know how you are thinking and working with them. Note too the possible significance of seemingly irrelevant tangential preoccupations and symptoms. In this way the history-taking and consultation becomes more of a shared learning experience by both doctor and patient with a meeting of minds rather than a divergence. The history is always a pointer to depths which the patient may or may not be aware of or has lost sight of. It is a guide-line to understanding and perspective and the doctor gives a new reality hope to the patient when he discusses the history as it emerges. A new and more accurate reality may emerge for the patient based on sharing and understanding as opposed to unreal, unlinked reassurance without a basis for it.

Just as the physical may be the outward manifestations of inner more psychological problems, so too the psychological — irritability, fear, anxiety or depression may be the inner signs of chronic physical difficulties. This sometimes occurs in long drawn-out problems like chronic catarrh, sinusitis, hay-fever, bronchitis, viral pneumonia, dysmenorrhoea or simply when the patient is worn down by a long-standing exhausting, seemingly incurable condition.

Always try to see the patient in terms of individual maturity and understanding. Any clinging to infantile-dependent states, unreal aims or goals either at work or in the home, may then be quite openly explored, discussed and their origins and reasons brought out into the open in a full and natural way — as part of the 'work' and history-taking. Any specific problem within the family area needs careful looking at to see if it is at all under-mining or causative to a present illness — reducing vitality, energy and resistance.

Note how frequently a physical illness has an early precursor stage within the mentals with jaded exhaustion, malaise or irritability — these deep psychological areas responding first to a particular stress situation attempting to contain and localise it. This avoids spill-over and early disturbances at a physical organ level with physical changes as a consequence.

Every patient is a person first and foremost and closeness and contact with that person — the inner self, hopes, goals, aspirations and inspirations is needed and should be part of the overall approach. Directions, aims or drives may at times seem lacking and a deep cause of disappointment, loneliness and isolation, with a sense of failure, of being lost, undirected, the personality presented as drifting and self-defeating. Such attitudes may be life-long with a trail of difficulties and previous failures, disappointments or broken relationships.

Independence and the capacity for work as well as pleasure is important in history-taking, especially the ability to admit some degree of vulnerability as well as need. Note also the presence and awareness of responsibility and self-role for what is happening — including the present problem or illness.

Where there is over-excitement, over-confidence and a general impression of living in elevated states of mind, such 'highs' are highly vulnerable, usually short-lasting states with probable underlying depressive problems. This may be denied and refuge taken in mood-swings rather than the facing up to and dealing with a particular difficulty or challenge.

Sexuality and problems in the intimate area are always important and need to be specifically asked about. Libido may be reduced in the young as much as in the elderly by business, pressure-living, constant travel and chronic jet-lag. Fast-food and alcohol usually add to the pressures and emphasises living on the 'outside' and in the immediate rather than at a more personal depth.

Case Report 1

A women aged 50, two years into her second marriage, came with chronic problems of backache, fatigue and depression. She was tense and anxious. It quickly emerged that all intimacy had ceased after 6 months of marriage and that her husband totally refused to discuss the problem with her. She felt that she had not achieved the standards he had expected from her and felt rebuffed and frustrated. She feared that any approach to him would both aggravate her own personal needs and feelings and only add to the problem. She had opted to stay distant from him in the hope of provoking his interest but without a result. All of this greatly increasing her tension and depression. Her constitutional *Pulsatilla* led to greatly increased confidence and openness which completely resolved the intimate problems and her depression.

Case Report 2

A happily married, successful business man came with problems of exhaustion, recurrent genital herpes and total loss of sexual interest, except when on holiday when he was 'normal'. Here the problem was of excessive work involvement and a refusal to delegate. Work was taken home in the evenings and at weekends. There was no break in communication or affection within the couple. With *Nux vomica* the herpes condition cleared quickly as well as the fatigue, and libido availability. There were no reality problems in the business area but until *Nux vomica* was given he was unable to separate himself from them, feeling 'swallowed up', unable to sleep, relax or to be available for physical involvement. The remedy helped him to dissociate more from the work area, to feel relaxed, free and a person again.

For others, libidinal drives are excessive, painful or inappropriate and as much a problem as their absence. Always take careful note of basic constitutional make-up, normal variations, the patterns and any changes in libidinal drives. They are particularly susceptible to the 'externals' as diet, alcohol, synthetic pharmaceuticals and hormones as well as the classic 'internals' – pressure, demand and pace.

No man is an island, a machine or static in any part of him but infinitely changing and different in attitudes and functioning, psychologically and physiologically throughout life. Allowance and understanding must be made for all of this — especially in such delicate areas as the intimate and libidinal.

Where a patient presents his or her problem as *only* psychological — always check carefully the physical areas. Similarly where a basic problem presents as purely physical, pay particular attention to the psychological aspects. In this way the homoeopath acts in the patient's best total interests and is in a position of balance for history-taking, as well as for prescribing.

Where there is an obvious and almost too simple tangible problem don't overlook the intangibles and if the person comes with one that is intangible, vague or too obviously psychological, then always first exclude any organic tangible cause from the diagnosis.

It is usually the tangible elements of the history that are first presented — because they are most superficial, but also because they have been prepared in the patient's mind as what the doctor most wants to hear and are most acceptable to him. Other, perhaps significant symptoms, even whole areas may be left out or played down because they seem irrelevant are 'not what the doctor wants to hear' — in case they provoke anger or annoyance. 'A doctor's time is precious' — we are taught at school or earlier and he must not be given trivial, useless, irrelevant information. Because of such infantile anxieties every patient tends to some degree to edit what he gives, and in this way edits both himself and the illness. It is basic in homoeopathy not to let this happen and to make allowance and correction for it in history-taking so that a less distorted picture of the patient may emerge and a more relevant accurate prescription then follow.

The need with every person is to try to ascertain a true totality of the individual as far as it can be perceived within the consultation framework. Essentials are very often given in true Freudian fashion as the patient is leaving. The patient apologises and says that they may not be important or strictly relevant to the problem. The homoeopath knows that they are often *very* important and that what is said in the opening and closing moments of the consultation can be very significant. Because of these human factors, reasonable flexibility of consultation time is necessary so that some extra time can be allowed where necessary.

It is important in history-taking that the doctor should come over as a person, a human being, not as an omnipotent god-like authoritarian figure inspiring fear and awe.

When his example in the consulting room is one of true humility, this enables the patient also to find his or her own humility and identity.

In consulting work generally there is a need for greater trust and respect between doctor and patient with a joint work-task of clarification and diagnosis to be developed. This makes for a *human* medicine rather than a computer-based inhuman one. Essentially it is part of the art of healing which, in every case, must somewhere embrace a meeting of minds — of two people attempting to conduct a situation where information, associations, contact, helps make the homoeopathic diagnosis and where change can occur. This gives the possibility of greater self-realisation and a climate for under-standing.

A case-history is an important factual affair but it is only a part of the overall contact and meeting, of the therapy, because treatment has already begun to some degree with the taking of the history. Its development and unfolding is inseparable from the development and unfolding of the patient — ultimately of the cure and freeing of the individual.

For this to occur, time is needed as well as patience, attention and a real interest by the physician for the patient as a person and individual. Non-judgemental attitudes by both patient and doctor alike facilitate clarification and unfolding with a real depth to it. A mutual willingness to listen creates a climate that best supports the remedy as well as ensuring accuracy of prescribing.

Chapter nine

The Homoeopathic
Consultation

Homoeopathy is not only about prescribing, not only about matching symptoms to those of a 'proving' picture — this is relatively easy with some experience. But homoeopathy is also an important aspect of holistic medicine with all that implies for understanding and an approach to the individual. More than prescribing principles — no matter how important and basic to the method, homoeopathy is about people. The diagnosis must include this as part of its totality — with not just the symptoms taken into account, but also that the basic method itself is suitable treatment for the particular person. If not, homoeopathy should not be recommended or only be used as a second line of support and defence using other methods when better indicated for the patient.

Homoeopathy is not a panacea, it has its limitations like any other form of treatment.

The major concern of homoeopathy is the *overall* viewpoint, the patient's well-being and what is best for him or her. This overall statement accepts the patient as a uniquely different and differing individual.

Homoeopathy works with a varying degree of success depending not only on the accuracy of the prescription but also the human, caring way in which the remedies are given. Homoeopathy in a busy clinic with a factory atmosphere and a brief pressurised consultation is a quite different therapeutic tool to one where time and care are available with unruffled attention — not just for a first consultation but also for the follow-ups.

Where the doctor does not pretend omnipotence and can acknowledge simplicity and ordinaryness, he enables the patient not to play the child either. In this way he encourages and supports the patients to be themselves.

The homoeopathic approach is one which emphasises communication and dialogue as basic to healing. This is not something created by the remedy but an attitude of mind which adds to and facilitates its action in depth and supports the unique homoeopathic action of freeing vital energy flow. Where the physician is open and straightforward, the patient too can be more straightforward with him or herself facilitating an openness of expression which helps the illness to be understood with greater clarity and facilitates cure.

Homoeopathy is a quite unique system of medicine, rarely sufficiently appreciated even by practitioners. In the highest potencies it can unlock, mobilise and resolve long-standing blocks, facilitating growth at every level — not just at a physical level but also within the personality. In this way the remedy-potency supports personal growth, insight development and maturation. In its highest dilutions it will give comfort to otherwise unsupportable states of anguish and pain — undecipherable areas where there are no certainties and where none of us know for sure.

Where diagnosis not only matches a remedy but also plumbs the depths for the correct level of dis-ease, the right potency facilitates elimination and flow overcoming blockage and speeding cure — the patient helped to an optimum degree. The remedy itself gives the latitude and breadth of the illness — sets the boundaries but only the potency gives the depth. When both are correct then a unique, accurate therapeutic medicine is available for the patient.

Chapter ten

Homoeopathic Prescribing

The principles of choosing a remedy and the general approach to the patient are the elements of homoeopathy, fundamental and inseparable from the method.

In order to prescribe there must be symptoms — otherwise a homoeopathic potency should not be given. There is only one exception to this rule, when a remedy is being given prophylactically. A nosode may be given to a symptom-free pregnant women in contact with rubella in the early weeks or an elderly emphysematous patient given *Influenzinum* where exposure to influenza could be dangerous in epidemic conditions. Similarly a mumps or measles nosode may be given at contact stage where there are no symptoms and where development of the disease is undesirable for a variety or reasons. *Arnica* may be given to prevent blood-loss, bruising or shock before either a dental extraction or surgical procedure and *Caulophyllum* is frequently prescribed in the last weeks of pregnancy to facilitate delivery and maximise uterine tone. But these are the exceptions and homoeopathy is based on an individual prescription for the individual patient-totality and not as in conventional practice, to suppress and eradicate. Where homoeopathic prescribing is based only on local pathological symptoms it may not give very good results. Basing the remedy on appearance and local pathology at best gives only temporary relief.

Polypharmacy, or the use of more than one remedy at a time is not recommended although in some continental countries it is standard. 'Hit and miss' tactics deny the whole point of the homoeopathic consultation, are rarely successful and tend to build up a chain of therapeutic failures or partial results which only lead to lack of confidence by patient and physician alike. Mixed prescribing has never been part of the homoeopathic approach since its origins and is an example of unhomoeopathic thinking applied to the method — keeping it superficial and ignoring the basic principles and potential of the treatment.

Without exception the basic homoeopathic aim is to stimulate inherent vitality within the patient and a gradual revival of essential intrinsic energies, resilience and resistance. Symptom-eradication or suppression is also unhomoeopathic and should play no part in the method which basically aims to rather encourage and support their appearance and production because they reflect a healthy positive response.

Note that homoeopathy gives a vitality which is totally natural, giving confidence to patients who sense that *their* body is responding rather than producing an artificial reaction to camoflage or cover up.

Multiple prescribing also carries the risks of neutralising a remedy that is well-chosen but where more time is needed for a response. In most cases there is no need for an additional medicine at the time and their use is usually due to inexperience with the method. Neither doctor nor patient really knows for certain which remedy has had the effect and the uncertainty perpetuates a tendency to re-prescribe in a similar manner.

In general only prescribe the same remedy in the single dose particularly with the high potencies but repeat more frequently the lower ones. The only exception is the acute crisis when 'high' potencies may be given hourly or even every 10 minutes until there is a vital response — for a period of up to 12 hours, especially where a lower potency has failed to evoke a response. For many the single dose of the well chosen potency is adequate even with an acute problem and hourly 'highs' are the exception rather than the rule.

At all times homoeopathy aims to support and foster balanced healthy functioning within the inherent constitution or terrain, supporting vitality and resistance, both physically as well as psychologically.

Basic to the homoeopathic method is prescribing on the totality of symptoms which form the key features and uniqueness of the case — the internal as much the external patterns.

Recipe, appearance-prescribing is unlikely to succeed or give more than a temporary lull and reassurance but without the consistent real improvement that is needed. The human factor should be a part of the *art* of every prescription dispensed, indeed of healing in general and a factor to be taken into account in every illness — whatever its depth or appearance. In every condition and sickness there are always some gains, however painful or perverse this seems and motivation as well as the reasons for a condition or disease need careful thought and assessment at all times — especially with long-standing chronic problems.

Rules For Prescribing

1 Only prescribe on the healthy vital response of the individual, the symptoms and reactions and for no other reason.

2 Always prescribe on the combination and totality of both mentals and physicals to ensure a most complete picture — whatever the stated complaint.

3 Precipitating factors need careful appraisal and attention— like the origins of a case, especially where a patient has never been well since a certain 'event' like vaccination or a specific illness. In such cases a remedy may be needed — usually after the constitutional, to 'cover' the line between the original injury or sensitivity and the onset of symptoms.

4 Family history is important, frequently giving the clue to a miasmic condition and often confirmation of it. Examples are tuberculosis in a parent or grandparent, a history of earlier contact without actual illness and where the overall picture 'fits' that of the specific nosode.

5 The modalities and specifics — the odd, rare and peculiar symptom often give the confirmation to an indicated remedy from the history.

6 Where confirmation is weak, absent or unclear, always base the prescription on the remedy which 'fits' the majority of symptoms, but not necessarily the totality. When one of the symptoms seems at variance with the chosen remedy — perhaps marked thirst when all other symptoms indicate *Pulsatilla*, it should be prescribed nevertheless in spite of the lack of 'total fit'.

Chapter eleven

On the Choice of Remedy

The remedy has but one sole function — to support and direct vital energy to the desired areas of specific treatment to be revitalised and balanced. It indicates the specifics of the treatment, its boundaries and areas where energy, elimination, flow — both mental and physical are required or needed. The specific pathways of action of each remedy naturally limit its range and action to some extent — even where a polycrest or remedy of multiple action is chosen. Each remedy has its own predominant area and range of physiological activity — as part of its intrinsic nature and this is clearly seen when it is taken undiluted or in toxic doses.

Examples of specific physiological pathways for some remedies are:

Lycopodium — lungs, bladder, stomach, mentals.

Phosphorus – blood and circulation, lungs, mentals, liver.

Belladonna – skin, throat, ears and mentals.

Bryonia – lungs, joints, intestines.

Every remedy has the natural ability to stimulate a reaction within its own specific sphere – originating within the mother-substance and defining its inherent pathways, range of reaction, vitality and stimulation.

In addition to supporting vital energy, the physician has a further aim – to facilitate for each individual, increased awareness, dialogue and maturity. Where feelings are severely blocked, so too is vital energy and only accurate treatment and removal of the psychological block facilitates vital communication, essential dialogue and optimum remedy activity. These are well-known common causative factors in disease and their treatment is not so different from giving support to other vital energy systems. Such psychological impasses block individual expression, spontaneity and vitality – the essential self, as much as any physical scar – and in some cases even more so. Freedom 'to be' and to express, is one definition of vital energy because suppression at a deep fundamental level from emotional causes may completely distort or prevent all essential vital expressions.

Chapter twelve

The First Prescription

As much as possible the first prescription should be the overall constitutional one that acts on the global total of psychological and physiological systems, encompassing the basic temperamental backcloth as well as the physical modalities, specific variations and modifying features.

The constitutional acts deeply provided there are no severe mechanical factors to block it from initiating vital energy movement. Properly prescribed, the constitutional acts deeply upon the whole and total psychological and physiological systems of the individual whatever the level or degree of stress imbalance.

Symptom-relief alone is un-homoeopathic in thinking and approach, deviating from its primary aim to support and strengthen both locally and overall. The constitutional strengthens because it brings about a freeing of energy flow and balance within essential communication and energy-carrying pathways. An absence of flow or elimination leads to stagnation, irritation and diminished reserves. The illness-response or symptoms are the body's attempts to overcome such problems and redress the balance by using every reserve and defence at its disposal. It is these attempts by the organism which may be externally experienced as intermittent symptoms — bouts of fever, weakness, spasm, inflammation or periodic exacerbation of symptoms.

Treatment at times of symptom-activity gives dynamic support, harmonising with the body's needs, because when symptoms are active, so too is innate vitality on the move and the remedy helps make these responses more effective when previously insufficiently strong to cure an underlying condition. Where underlying dynamics are not clearly seen, the constitutional profile vague or unclear, it is often best to wait for a time and to do nothing, re-taking the history and re-assessing any possible remedy at the next visit.

Where this is impossible and some form of treatment needs to be started without delay, a nosode may be given to *clear* the underlying physiological terrain so that the appropriate pathway of dynamic activity can be more clearly seen and prescribed for. This is particularly important in chronic, long-standing cases where the vagueness and confusion are due to miasmic factors.

Other cases may be confused for different reasons. A variety of treatments in the past, including well-meaning self-help recipes may not have helped and even pushed underlying dynamics deeper. Suppressant synthetics frequently alter the picture of the dynamics without a positive healing effect on the overall problem. The relevant picture and area of struggle may be obscured to an extent which confuses both doctor and patient and accurate prescribing is impossible. *Sulphur* often stimulates a return of symptoms, throwing out the suppressants from other interventions so that effective prescribing and treatment can be commenced again.

When prescribing a first constitutional always observe and record any specific symptoms of the patient — especially anything strange, odd, localised, or at all bizarre. This may give the clue to the next remedy as well as pin-pointing the areas of activity as vague, general and unsatisfactory symptoms disappear to give way to more clear-cut reactions and indications for prescribing.

Examples Of Specifics, and Peculiar Diagnostic Symptoms For Remedies

1 Swelling of the upper eyelids
   — *Kali carb*

2 Flapping of the nasal wings when breathing
   — *Lycopodium*

3 One foot hot, the other cold
   — *Lycopodium*

4 The body feels as if made of glass or containing a live animal
   — *Thuja*

5 There is loss of bowel control leading to incontinence when emotionally excited
   — *Hyoscyamus*

Chapter thirteen

The Second Prescription

This follows up the first, what is clarified by it and is in need of further treatment. The homoeopathic potency 'pushes out' the remains of any blockages or suppressed long-standing problems — back into the body's active defensive layers to be more 'available' and amenable to its actions. In this way imbalance can be effectively harmonised and resolved. Deeper physical symptoms, may also be 'released' by the remedy as previously non-functioning physical or psychological areas are activated again by the developing dynamic process and homoeopathic potency.

Making non-functioning areas more effective supports their balance and integration into the total, but sometimes experienced as *new* surface symptoms or a *return* of previous patterns and problems — not felt for some time. An attitude of depression and irritability may be replaced by an arthritic problem which has been quiescent for months. This making more superficial and 'available' is key to homoeopathy and reflects a major response to the remedies. The body's natural defensive energy can then get to grips with the *dynamised* blockages and either neutralise or stimulate them to more balanced vitality again.

The remedy itself does not neutralise an imbalance — this it cannot do. But by supporting natural innate channels of vitality it allows a blocked abnormal pattern to be lifted from the shadow of a physiological impasse into the light of day. All this activity is shown externally by one event only — the aggravation or reaction to the remedy and the appearance of symptoms expressing vital reaction taking its course and curative direction.

Partial improvement followed by a relapse, always suggests a possible underlying mechanical problem or obstruction. This may require surgical correction before any potency can act or be complete.

The remedy itself may also be incorrect or ineffective. But in all cases whenever there is temporary relief only and no true aggravation followed by improvement, it is important to consider the diagnosis of possible organic problems with permanent blockage to vitality, flow and functioning. Such mechanical problems may sometimes respond and clear with homoeopathy but often they are the result of long-standing disturbances — not treated sufficiently early and vital energy in the area is minimal. In such cases homoeopathy may be best as a second line of treatment because of irreversible changes. These cases often need surgery and only after correction can homoeopathy be really effective. It is important not to delay an effective operative treatment by trying to apply homoeopathy where it is not most indicated.

When the first constitutional or clarifying remedy has been successful, it is usual for symptoms to emerge more clearly and with greater force than before. This is because there is now a meaning and logic to them because of the remedy's action which the patient reflects by increased vitality. The roots and origin of the whole illness may now emerge much more comprehensibly as they link to form a more meaningful whole.

After the initial prescription it is classical to do nothing and 'wait and see'. As long as the patient is improving and 'better' the physician should not re-prescribe, interrupt or interfere with the mobilising and the freeing process.

Indications For a Second Prescription

1 There has been no improvement from the first, the patient feeling worse as a result with new symptoms developing. In such cases it is best to neutralise the first remedy and re-take the history, the new symptoms indicating a new and different remedy.

2 Where new symptoms occur, either physical or psychological and overwhelm the patient with little general increase in well-being — re-prescribe to encompass the new areas and symptoms released.

3 When new material or new symptoms released relate to earlier forgotten complaints of relevance to the origins of the present condition, it may be urgent to treat them as soon as possible. As a result of the first constitutional a dry cough resembling an earlier TB infection may occur or the patient develop evening sweats with loss of weight. In such cases it is important to give the nosode early rather than delay — but depending always upon the individual and the judgement of the doctor. In every case the individuality of the patient takes priority over every other consideration especially theoretical concepts and ideals.

4 Where new symptoms occur as a result of the first prescription, but the patient is generally better, do not re-prescribe. Wait

always until improvement has slowed down markedly or stopped. Exactly when to re-prescribe when there is a slowing down of improvement and progress is a question of clinical judgement and skill, dependent upon the merits of the individual case and overall picture. If all improvement has totally ceased after a period of fairly consistent gains then it is usual to re-prescribe according to the symptom-picture of that time.

5 Where there has been an aggravation not followed by improvement and there has been no true 'healing' crisis, it is usual to prescribe again on the basis of the total symptom-pattern of the time and not on the previous history or earlier profiles.

6 When there is an organic condition like angina or hypertension with underlying 'wear and tear' to the constitution, the patient generally improved by the remedy, but the angina and blood-pressure remaining unchanged or still critical, it may be advisable to re-prescribe. This is usually best in low potency — either a 3x or 6c — because these symptoms represent a danger to the patient until they have had time to lessen and diminish. In every case without exception, it is the patient who matters — whatever the principles of a method — even homoeopathic ones. Every case, every step and every prescription must *only* be based on the individual needs at the time and the

judgement of the physician — nothing else matters.

7   Re-prescribe when there is no improvement, sense of well-being, general energy release, sleep amelioration or lessening of tension as a result of the initial prescription.

8   Where the improvement is sluggish, weak, or short-lasting as to be almost negligible, the symptom-picture remaining essentially the same, repeat the same initial remedy. If necessary repeat in higher potency until there is an aggravation and response.

In *Lectures on Homoeopathic Philosophy*, Kent clearly states that the second prescription should only be a meaningful extension of the first and nothing else. He stressed that the first prescription should only be changed when there is a good reason to do so but for none other. He emphasises that a second potency should not be administered too soon after the first or until it has had sufficient time to produce similar symptoms to the original illness in one form or other and some expression of vital reaction which gives the clearest indications for a possible second prescription.

In general he recommends a second potency only after there has been no further movement or reaction from a first and where change is at a standstill. When the original symptoms recur after a first potency, changed or modified in some way — perhaps increased or retarded, he sees this as the optimum criteria of a positive response. If the original symptoms complained of become less frequent, less intense, this is also taken as an encouraging positive sign of a 'like' cure. In such cases, emphasises Kent, the second prescription should be one and one only — a repeat of the first, once all change and improvement has ceased.

After a first prescription, wait for a return of the symptom-image which emerges when the first remedy has exhausted its action and until there is a cure. In this way we can know if it was deep enough or just a superficial remedy. General improvement of the patient is a positive sign. An aggravation with some decline of the patient's well-being is doubtful. If the patient is 'better' it may be too generalised and apply to just a few symptoms. Only a generalised total improvement is a real indication of cure. If the patient is not generally better overall, then trivial superficial apparent improvements may indicate a negative outcome rather than an improved positive one.

Every symptom is the expression of debility of the patient as well as his or her vital reaction and attempts at resolution and cure.

Once the curative impulse has subsided, symptoms always re-appear as an overall profile of the present illness position which is the very best basis for further prescribing. Only represcribe a second potency when the first has been fully completed so that the emergent symptoms re-constitute a picture which can be relied upon. If not — wait. If the prescription given was the simillimum and a correct one, the symptoms which return will be the same and confirm the need for the same remedy. Even in chronic disease continue the same remedy as long as the returning symptom-image is the same as the original. If the same remedy fails to stimulate a positive curative response, then give it in higher potency.

When symptoms come back slightly changed with the absence of some of the original features but none which are new, the remedy should not be changed.

In every case make a trial of the highest potencies of a well-indicated remedy when a lower one has not evoked a satisfactory response.

The key to a second prescription is one only — the appearance of new symptoms — the only indication for a new or different remedy. The first prescription is made from the entire total image of the sickness and matched against the remedy profile to find the simillimum remedy. If this first prescription has not been well chosen, it may be necessary to make a second as a result of error at that time.

If the first prescription causes symptoms to become deeper, the patient worse, antidote at once. When an antidote is not known, the new symptoms must be prescribed for as a totality.

In incurable disease when an inappropriate or a wrong remedy has stimulated destructive symptoms, also antidote immediately.

Where the general state of the patient is worsening, the first prescription may have been a partial one only and not a total fit for the patient and the true simillimum, or the disease is in-curable. In incurable cases, a second pre-scription should be given for any new suffering as it occurs but in low potencies unless terminal when a higher potency gives relief and tranquillity with peace of mind.

If new symptoms occur yet the disease is perfectly curable, it is likely that the first remedy was inaccurate and not the patient's true simillimum.

The greatest hazard in homoeopathy is to follow prescription upon prescription based on the smallest trivial changes and repeated too frequently. Symptoms that emerge after the first and their *direction* of change is the basis for assessing each subsequent prescription, whether the patient is generally better or not. The first prescription aims to set in motion vital energy movement in a direction favourable for the re-establishment of equilibrium and this should never be interfered with until exhausted. The second has a close positive supportive relationship to the first and should be in concordance with it.

In chronic states the remedy that best conforms to the acute illness is important to keep in mind, as often the 'chronic' of that remedy is the one most needed and indicated.

The Following Have Complementry Relationships.

Calcarea in the chronic of *Belladonna* and *Rhus tox.*

Natrum mur is the chronic of *Apis* and *Ignatia*

Silicea is the chronic of *Pulsatilla*

Sulphur is the chronic of *Aconitum.*

The Following Remedies Have an Antagonistic Relationship to Each Other:

Causticum and *Phosphorus*

Apis and *Rhus tox.*

In summary, the greatest pitfall of every second prescription is either to prescribe too low in potency, or there is an inability to wait until the first has exhausted itself. Patient caution and time are always of major importance in prescribing, especially after a previous 'high' first prescription.

Summary Of The Major Indications For a Second Prescription

1 Where there is a new tendency developing with new symptoms of a different type from those previously complained of, the remedy needs to be antidoted, its action stopped and a new prescription given.

2 Sometimes it is necessary to add to and complement a first prescription. An acute treatment may have been given for an acute condition as *Belladonna* for scarlet fever or *Rhus Tox* for shingles, the specific nosode for glandular fever. In such cases it may be necessary to follow the specific by a constitutional to support a slow convalescence with perhaps vulnerability to future infection and illness.

3 Where the first constitutional throws up old symptoms of a long-since forgotten illness — a previous gonorrhoea — the patient never well since that time, or in others following whooping cough, vaccination, virus pneumonia or typhoid, prescribe either a nosode or a specific remedy.

On The Danger Of Prescribing On Appearance Only And Not On The Totality

In every case, symptoms heal from above downwards, from deeper to more superficial, and in reverse order of origin and first appearance (Hering's Law).

Where a deeper problem has improved — as breathlessness on climbing stairs with swelling of ankles, or angina of effort replaced by more superficial problems — as arthritic pain in the shoulder or hip, it is a mistake to rush in and treat these new symptoms in isolation, ignoring their deeper meaning. These more peripheral symptoms usually resolve quite spontaneously with the same prescription — given time and as long as a patient is improving. No additional outside help from a further remedy or treatment is required as the body can usually deal with them itself once vitality and energy flow is re-established.

Case History

A woman of 50 came with angina of effort and raised blood-pressure. After an initial prescription she was much improved and her chest pain, racing pulse and palpitations were almost negligible. She complained however that she was not better because she had developed a recurrence of an old problem — arthritis in the right hip and that her periods were now prolonged and heavier. In every other way she felt markedly better however. Note that arthritis is a more superficial symptom than a cardiac one and that the uterus is a peripheral organ to the heart. Vital energy blockage had very positively shifted from a deeper organ to a more superficial one, at the same time throwing up an old recurrent, unresolved problem that she had not felt for some years. It was explained that this was a very favourable positive hom-oeopathic response and that there were no indications to change her remedy or treatment because the original prescription was still working and that if not interrupted or inter-fered with, she was likely to further improve. The patient was relieved and reassured and at her next visit reported a lessening of both the hip discomfort and her menstrual problems.

Chapter fourteen

Subsequent Prescribing

This must always be directed at the overall picture rather than at any symptom-relief only. As long as there is an improvement do not change or alter the prescription in any way or repeat. If low potencies are being taken they should be stopped as soon as symptom-relief occurs and the patient have specific instructions to this effect.

At all times guage the depth and level of a problem as well as its more lateral planes and outward manifestations, prescribing accordingly. For a 'tangible', obvious, palpable problem of relatively superficial level, give the low 3x or 6c 'tangible' potency. Where a deeper problem exists, give a 30c at least and for chronic or psychological levels of disturbances, give a 200c. Try always to prescribe as accurately for the level as well as the outer manifestations and in every consultation, clarify the depths — the tangibles as well as intangibles, in order to ascertain the most accurate remedy. Try not only to make an illness-diagnosis but as much as possible also complement and complete the patient's own picture and understanding of his or her illness. In this way the best psychological 'soil' or attitudes for the patient are created giving optimum support to the eventual potencies prescribed.

In general subsequent prescriptions should relate only to any new emergent patterns of symptoms as they occur or where former problems have not responded. When there has been no response, or only minimal gains by the patient, a fresh potency from a new source should be considered when the remedy seems well-indicated. Alternatively increase the potency up the scale, provided that the clinical picture still indicates it.

In general and with minor exceptions only, prescribe once only and then wait and see. Clarke in *The Prescriber* recommends that where there has been no response to a seemingly well-indicated remedy, that it should be repeated at more frequent intervals until a vital reaction occurs. Subsequently the doctor must wait until this response is exhausted before giving another remedy and for as long as the same symptoms keeps returning. If a different set of symptoms occurs — he recommends re-prescribing with a new remedy unless they relate to early, once suppressed symptoms and the patient is generally improved when nothing should be done or changed.

Chapter fifteen

Modalities

These are the highly individual constitutional variations which play such a key role in every homoeopathic assessment of the individual and in the choice of remedy. They relate to major areas of physiological functioning, especially energy reserve, circulation, distribution and conservation, as temperature regulation and heat control of the body. The resilience and response to outer physical factors and pressures as well as to internal ones and the ability to deal and constantly adjust to change is what ultimately makes for health and individuality. This must always be assessed in the choice and confirmation of each remedy.

Identical twins may both develop a throat infection at the same time but there is no certainty that each will respond in the same way or need the same remedy. They are likely to show quite distinct responses − both physically as well as psychologically. One is gasping for air, screaming for the window to be left wide open and in floods of angry tears if delayed (*Pulsatilla*). The other is sensitive to the least draught of cool air and considerably worse for an open window with a fussy withdrawal and demands for extra layers of clothes rather than tears (*Arsenicum*). Each clearly requires a different remedy for effective prescribing and is differentiated by the modalities and symptoms.

Every physiological terrain or background is unique — even with identical twins. Each has individual strengths or weakness according to temperament, constitution, physiological and hereditary factors. The modalities tend to be constant once maturity has been reached and may be the only clue to the correct prescription when the overall symptom-profile is not decisive. The modality-factors include reactions to heat, chill, dryness, humidity, fatigue and when most energy is released — morning or later in the day, or the time of an energy 'low'. Exposure to environmental externals particularly heat as much as cold can be dangerous particularly for anyone debilitated, after acute illness or when convalescent. or weak from an unusual physical effort — the body not cooled down sufficiently before exposure to heat as taking a hot shower or sauna. When fasting with rapid weight-loss over a short period, with exhaustion and weakness is followed by exposure to heat, there may be the risk of heart or circulatory problems when the person is susceptible. One patient developed angina of effort, having been perfectly fit before a fast, After lying in the hot sun all summer in a depleted exhausted state, she quickly developed heart weakness, angina and circulatory insufficiency.

Often the modalities are internal ones and reflect intolerance, anger, impatience, frustration or the inability to accept a situation of not knowing. Each is a threat in some way to security and needs assessing as part of the mentals or psychological profile for the modalities and the individuality implications.

One patient may be better for rain (*Ruta*), another aggravated by it (*Rhus tox*) or by changes — of weather or atmospherics (*Dulcamara*) or from a storm (*Rhododendron*). A patient may be relieved by thunder (*Sepia*) or over-sensitive to it (*Phosphorus*). Many are worse for heat and quite unable to tolerate it (*Pulsatilla, Argentum nitricum*), yet others are better for heat and crave warmth (*Arsenicum, Calcarea*). Many are in need of constant attention, concern and reassurance (*Lycopodium, Phosphorus*). Others want to be left alone and are aggravated by too much attention and resent it (*Natrum mur, Sepia*).

In this way a profile to complement as well as confirm the symptom profile is established so that a remedy emerges which 'fits' in as many areas as possible, based on both the unique psychological as well as physiological patterns and responses, giving the individualisation which is so essential and unique to homoeopathy.

Chapter sixteen

Prescribing for Acute Problems

Where problems are tangible, acute and clear-cut, give the 6th centesimal potency, or similar 'low' potency frequently – if necessary every few minutes until relief occurs. When less acute, give hourly. Use the higher potency only if clearly indicated and then do not repeat as frequently as a 'low' one – but according to judgement, the individual case and the response. A 30th potency should not generally be used for acute cases unless it is the only potency available and then give hourly only. If there is little or no response with the 6c potency, change to a highter potency of the same remedy, but always observe the responses to a single dose.

Homoeopathy will not work at all completely if acute symptoms are the result of a foreign body, acute blockage, obstruction, displacement, or dislocation. These need to be urgently adjusted, corrected or treated by an appropriate physical approach related to their cause and the under-lying problems of the patient.

As the patient improves – following any aggravation, provided there is sufficient available vital energy, stop the remedy and observe. In every acute case the patient is in a crisis of elimination with inability to externalise and excrete an internal irritant due to blockage or stasis of drainage of the acute condition. Homoeopathy supports and facilitates this drainage, allowing energy to flow again, always provided that it is not of mechanical origin. Every related potency facilitates such movement, energy distribution and a return to healthy functioning.

In each acute case – as throughout homoeopathy, the acute prescription must only be prescribed on the totality of individual presenting symptoms and not on pathology or any diagnostic label. Give the specific nosode e.g. *Influenzinum* for influenza, once only in an acute epidemic condition when indicated or if the vital response to the indicated remedy is weak, delayed or in any way unsatisfactory.

Chapter seventeen

Prescribing for Chronic Problems

These are the most difficult of all to treat because vital response is inevitably sluggish and minimal. There is usually a long-term crisis associated with intoxication and stasis of some kind with a slowing down generally of physiological responses and a failure to eliminate over a prolonged period. The body lacks the strength to achieve an acute healing aggravation or significant vital response so that there can be no quick or easy resolution by the patient of the typical blockage and stasis.

When a case is irreversible, it lacks sufficient drive, vitality and energy to eliminate internal irritating barriers and to bring them to resolution — either from physical or psychological reasons. It remains incurable and chronic within the system until a change occurs in the availability of vital response to the area affected. Where the problem is irreversible, the cure left too late, the prescription should be kept to the lower 3x/6c potencies and it is an error to prescribe 'high'. Such prescribing may evoke a violent reaction — even a fatal one and it is only indicated for terminal suffering, when it is very valuable to ease anguish and to bring peace of mind, with awareness at a maximum and analgesics kept minimal.

In chronic illness, more than with acute problems, the aim is to restore balanced vital functioning and circulation to the area affected — physiologically and psychologically as part of the essential stimulus needed. The aim is improved function and flow, a healthier physiological 'soil' overcoming stagnation and retention with optimum stimulation of elimination and drainage which is key to overcoming every chronic state.

Chronic problems inevitably mean blockage, failure of flow and lack of detoxication so that essential drainage is always a prime aim of the homoeopathic intervention. Once there is a return to the homoeopathic aggravation, there is equally a return to vitality and an overcoming of any poverty of flow or suppression to underlying dynamics. In the past there may have been minor peaks or exacerbations of symptoms, but no true aggravation and in this way the system retained its same position of stasis over a prolonged period. Because of this stasis there could be no spontaneous cure.

In chronic conditions a miasm must always be considered and a specific anti-miasmic remedy given at an early stage in treatment where an indicated potency fails to evoke a satisfactory response. It should not then be repeated for at least several months after the prescription and in this way resembles nosode-prescribing.

Chapter eighteen

'Proving' a Remedy

This may happen where there is sensitivity to a
remedy — occuring usually only when it has
been given over a prolonged period, either in
'low' or unnecessary 'high' potency beyond the
period of symptom-recovery. If severe, the
remedy should be stopped immediately and if
there is no lessening of proving-symptoms, the
remedy neutralised to eliminate it from the
system. Such symptoms are different from a
positive aggravation and it is important always
to be able to differentiate a proving sensitivity-
reaction from the emergence of new symptoms,
or a worsening of the original condition.

Case-Example Of 'Proving' A Remedy

A patient had been taking *Arnica* 6 daily on a
self-prescribed basis for fatigue over several
weeks. After 10 days he was considerable better
but against all homoeopathic principles, he
decided to continue on with the remedy because
he felt so well. After 3 weeks an intense
localised, left-sided chest discomfort developed

in the inter-costal muscles that nothing would relieve. The pain was of a severe bruised nature — as if he had been kicked. This pain was identical with the proving profile of *Arnica*. All symptoms were better for lying on the side, for support and for generally immobilising the area. The bed felt unusually hard and uncomfortable. On stopping *Arnica* all symptoms disappeared within 24 hours.

Chapter nineteen

The Homoeopathic Aggravation

This may occur with every well-prescribed remedy and represents a change in the internal dynamics of the case as improvement occurs. Some change or movement of symptoms *must* occur somewhere for a cure to take place, representing a new movement of vitality in the areas affected. It is usually mild and the patient does not lose any new-found sense of well-being and relaxation. Commonest is a change in the intensity of major symptoms or a worsening of the clinical state. Temporary in nature and lasting from a few up to 48 hours, it is more prolonged in chronic states and least following an acute illness. Aggravation is specifically provoked by the remedy and means that it is working according to homoeopathic plan and intention. Pathological patterns inherent within the remedy's make-up need to be just a little stronger than the underlying 'similar' disease pattern of the patient. The aggravation which the patient experiences is a healthy indication that this desired interaction is occuring.

In acute disease the initial aggravation is typically short and sharp, indicating a pathology which is 'available' and relatively on the surface for the homoeopathic stimulus to bring back into balance and vitality.

In chronic disease aggravation is much less well-defined, more vague and general — like the symptoms themselves. When chronic symptoms become worse, this is usually positive for the patient and aimed for, indicating no further interference with the last remedy, at least for the time being.

Chapter twenty

Miasms

These are the inherited, attenuated forms of earlier disease-patterns recurring in subsequent generations. They carry over the traces of previous severe diseases like T.B., syphilis, through other members of the family and may date from the remote past. A miasmic condition is different from the original 'mother' disease and pathology. There is no organ or tissue damage as occurred in the original disease yet it retains sufficient of these characteristics to clearly indicate its roots and origins. Miasms and their understanding are particularly important in chronic disease and are responsible for many recurrent and seemingly interminable problems of mankind.

In most cases the miasmic thread manifests as an undermining irritation to the expression and flow of ideas, energy, drive and vitality affecting every organ of the body in some way, to lessen health and well-being. Hahnemann grouped the major miasms under the following headings:

Psora: suppressed scabies or 'itch' is now most commonly seen as psoriasis.

Sycosis: suppressed gonorrhoea — now most commonly occurs as genital herpes and a wide variety of chronic inflammatory recurrent joint or urinary symptoms.

Syphilis: suppressed syphilis, manifests as changed or stunted mental and physical growth, arteriosclerosis, premature degeneration and aging.

Chapter twenty-one

The Choice and Function of Homoeopathic Potency

Potency relates directly to the depth of prescribing and should always be accurately plumbed during each consultation to determine the depth of the impaired functioning so that it can be treated at an optimum level. Every consultation should aim to decipher and correct energy blockages and at what levels there is distortion and disturbance. This may be superficial, at tissue level, intermediate, with mixed organ and tissue involvement, or deep with acute or chronic psychological problems, constitutional or inspirational disturbances. The deepest levels are most associated with overspill into the physical, as occurs in ulcerative colitis, peptic ulcer and asthma.

Low Potencies (3x - 12c)

These act on the most tangible conditions at tissue and cellular levels with a problem which is obvious, physical, measurable and palpable, clearly marked as to pathology — that 'something' is wrong and where. A common example might be a boil, cut, black-eye or a bruise. The prescription is repeated until there is a healthy aggravation or a definite improvement of the condition.

It is ideally suited for localised conditions, particularly where damage, trauma, or an inflammatory - irritant or allergic manifestation is obvious and definable. Other examples are haematoma or the accumulation of blood, a localised swelling after a sting or animal bite, indeed for any condition of limited damage and irritation to local tissues, nerves, tendons, veins or muscle. The more tangible the problem, the more tangible or lower is the potency required. In acute, tender prolapsed haemorrhoids, the chosen remedy, perhaps *Aloes* or *Hamamelis* is prescibed on appearance, site, modalities, history and variability but the potency is solely chosen on the depth of disturbance. The remedy here could equally have been *Pulsatilla*, *Lachesis*, *Belladonna* or *Sulphur* each having its specific clinical picture and indications. Where the acute problem is a prolapsed pile alone then the 6c potency is sufficient. But where the condition is also associated with deeper feelings like depression, then give the 30c potency which has greater penetration and needs to be given far less frequently then a lower dilution. In an acute tangible external problem, give the 3x potency hourly until there is a response. A 6c potency can equally be given hourly throughout the day in an acute condition but it is more usual to give 2-hourly. Always in homoeopathy it is the overall condition of the individual pattern that decides the potency, frequency of dosage and the remedy, and not any recipe-principles or dogma. Normally a 6c potency is given 3 times daily, possible 4 times until there is marked improvement when the potency can be stopped and a waiting period of observation given without the remedy to confirm that improvement is maintained and that no other remedy or potency is needed.

Where there is uncertainty, give the 3x potency for clear-cut obvious conditions with no known psychological associations. Give the 6c potency where a condition is localised but with more anxiety and restlessness although the major precipitating cause is not psychological and the needs for comfort, reassurance, and any fear or anxiety reactions are secondary only to the immediate shock or a fall. Consider the 30c potency when the problem is more repetitive, possibly with deep-seated psychological factors as with accident-proneness.

Middle Potencies (30c)

These intermediate dilutions are indicated for more mixed physical and psychological problems where the latter can be clearly seen. A common example is the adult or child who is repeatedly accident-prone at times of stress — before an examination, or where finalising end-of-year office figures, adds further to existing high levels of pressure. Another example might be irritability or psychological holding-in generally, with withdrawal and failure to communicate combined with constipation, indigestion or lack of energy. The potency is generally given 3 times weekly because as potency is increased, so too the life and range of the remedy is prolonged as well as deepened. In general use, the 30c potency is the ideal where psychological factors like anxiety, fear, insecurity and depression are marked but also associated with definite physical problems needing treatment, as obesity, constipation, indigestion, eczema, 'low-back', asthma, diarrhoea, rheumatism. It is an important potency that combines an equally balanced approach to the physical as well as the mentals. The 30c potency emphasises body areas, organs and physiological functions as well as the mentals and psychological processes provided that these are not overwhelming to the patient. It is ideal for home use and the family medicine chest.

High Potencies (200-10 M and above)

These should be given once only and not re-peated without clear-cut instructions to re-prescribe. The exception is certain very acute constitutional cases and then only in a crisis and for the briefest possible time until there is vital response and resolution. Clarification of its effects is essential and a single dose is usually adequate if given sufficient time to evoke a response, provided that the remedy is well-chosen and a good match to the patient's predominant symptoms. The single remedy is often quite enough to initiate a curative re-sponse from which all therapy can logically pro-ceed — either with or sometimes without any further interference. The emergent patterns and any new developments are then assessed as to whether a further potency is required.

High potencies are only recommended in general for the deepest constitutional chronic problems. Their activity and life varies with the remedy chosen but can be from 4 to 12 weeks or longer. They should only be re-prescribed after all improvement has ceased or there has been no response. Such 'high' repeats should always be given as infrequently as possible. Where a nosode has been prescribed it is inadvisable to repeat before 6 months and then only if strictly necessary and indicated.

Clarke states in *The Prescriber* that every potency can be curative provided the remedy is accurate and correct but the highest potencies

114

are most permanent in their cure. I understand him to mean – most radical, deep and complete in action.

In general high potencies are only indicated for chronic conditions, miasmic problems, and as the patient's constitutional in clinical work. Also where there is a specific indication, as a nosode following exposure to tuberculosis, or after glandular fever, scarlet fever, diptheria. They are also indicated where the prescriber is moving up the potency scale and a lower, well-chosen potency - eg 30c, has not evoked sufficient vital response and healing. It is generally recommended for every aspect of con-stitutional prescribing and preventative work, vaccination-reactions and vaccination-illness. In deep-seated psychological states, as mania, phobia, psychosis, it is essential to prescribe 'high' in order to provoke a profound response. With traumatic illness – as after head injury, exposure to acute fear or any injury, recent or remote – even one that occurred many years ago and led to a chronic condition, always pre-scribe 'high'. Where health and functioning are severely under-mined, then a 'high' potency is usually the first essential prescription to start the long road back to health and recovery.

High potencies generally provoke and stimu-late healthy organ activity and re-functioning and have an important role to play in problems of toxic elimination and chronic devitalised states.

In conclusion, the following principles apply to the choice of potency in general:

1 The clearer the mental involvement, the higher the potency.

2 The clearer the physical picture, but where the mentals are less significant, absent or obscure, prescribe 'low' except for chronic constitutional disorders.

3 In physical conditions without obvious clear-cut causes but a well-balanced, previously healthy personality, prescribe 'low'.

Chapter twenty-two

Organ Remedies

This is a related approach to illness where
specific remedies are given in homoeopathic
potency for specific organs or regions of the
body. The major organ prescribers include
Rademacher and Burnett. The latter in his —
Diseases of the Spleen (1887) stated that organ
prescribing or 'organopathy' with its emphasis
on organ pathology and organ remedies is a
concept upon which homoeopathy is based and
a wider extension to it. Burnett lists specific
remedies for the spleen including *Caenothus
americanus, Carco veg, Squilla, Quercus glan-
dium spiritus, Juniperus communis, Conium
mac* and others. For Burnett a remedy like
Cantharis is basically a kidney organ remedy,
Digitalis a heart remedy and *Belladonna* an
artery or circulation remedy. But to prescribe
Belladonna only on the grounds of palpitations
and thumping of the heart is to considerably
limit its range and importance as a constitutional remedy. In a similar way to prescribe *Caenothus americanus* for upper left-
sided abdominal pain and *Chelidonium* for

upper right-sided similar symptoms is to lessen and over-simplify homoeopathy and the very considerable depth and range of its remedies.

There is still a tendency to try to make homoeopathy easy and 'pathological' by thinking that *Arnica* is only a remedy for bruises and trauma, *Rhus tox* is *the* remedy for rheumatism, *Pulsatilla* only a female remedy, *Chamonilla* predominantly and only a children's remedy for teething. Such thinking is not so different from the 'organ approach' and the true range of the remedies is in danger of becoming limited and lessened. Some remedies do have particular or predominant action on an organ or side of the body but in the proving pictures upon which homoeopathy is based, it is always the overall totality of the picture which gives the remedy its range, shape and emphasis rather than any one localised activity. As Dr Marjorie Blackie made clear in her book — *The Patient, Not The Cure,* in homoeopathy the emphasis is upon the individual and his or her overall uniqueness, rather than any pathology or particular diseased organ which is the end-result and not the cause of disease. To prescribe on outcome and results rather than on causation is to miss the whole point of the homoeopathic approach and the depth of the method. A remedy in highest potency can unlock a cause going back not just several years but sometimes several generations and this is of inestimable value to the patient.

Where an 'organ' remedy fits the patient overall as *Pulsatilla* might constitutionally a patient with fluid retention problems, or *Phosphorus, a* chronic liver problem, *Sepia* a woman with chronic uterine problems, then there is no problem. To prescribe for the overall totality is in soundest homoeopathic traditions, in keeping with modern viewpoints and the very best interest of the patient.

In general there is little to be gained by prescribing an 'organ' remedy unless it fits the totality — when it is no longer an 'organ' remedy but one in keeping with the patient's overall make-up.

Chapter twenty-three

The Clinical Grid

The clinical grid can be used to plot treatment progress and outcome on simple graph paper. Use 10 squares to the inch and the following parameters to guage change and direction of response as a result of the homoeopathic potency. In general I have found it best to use a 10 point scale, set 1" apart on the graph paper.

The grid aims to give a reliable and accurate guage of change from the homoeopathic intervention, as well as a measure of its direction and a guide to prognosis for the patient. It is convenient and easy to record, giving an up-to-date measure of constitutional well-being and psychological health as well as the degree to which either the physical or the psychological factors dominate, distort or over-whelm the other.

The parameters can be varied considerably by the physician according to the patient's individual needs and profile, but once decided upon, must be kept constant for the duration of the treatment and as long as the grid is being recorded. For accuracy and completeness they include a measure of both the mentals and physical aspects of the patient. Both are inseparable and basic to the homoeopathic diagnosis, to prescribing and for patient-assessment whatever the complaints, and cannot be ignored.

For reasons of logic and simplicity, I have tried to keep the psychological parameters in the upper horizontal part of the grid and the physicals in the lower vertical parameters but this could be varied and whatever is decided, it is important to be consistent.

I have found the following psychological parameters to be most generally useful in my own clinical work and from experience with trying various alternatives. The parameters *dialogue, openness, sharing, communication* measured on a 10 point scale cover the major psychological areas of relationship, inter-change and constitution.

When assessing the physical parameters, I usually begin with the following and only vary them if necessary and where it is appropriate for a particular case or set of symptoms. The ones I use most commonly are the parameters: *Physical well-being, vitality and energy-availability*

The Grid In Clinical Practice

The following give some examples of the working value of the grid and its possible application and use for other physicians.

When beginning I assess the most appropriate points for each patient. The Physical Point is often immediately clear from the history and can be plotted at once. The Psychological Point takes a little experience but is not different and either emerges from the history, or is clearly seen in the consulting room from the degree of rapport and contact in the doctor-patient relationship and confirmed or otherwise by relatives and family where relevant. The midpoint of a line joining both Physical and Psychological points gives the first 'Constitutional' point X for the patient as in Diagram 1 — which is more fixed and less mobile than the second 'Symptom' point.

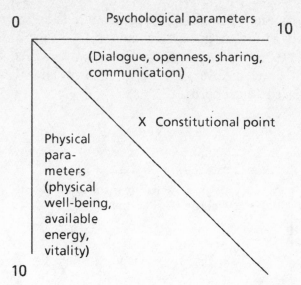

Diagram 1

The second Symptom point is formed by plotting, this time on a single transverse parameter, the individual patient-responses and symptom-dynamics of the case but always including both mentals and physicals. This point 0 gives a measure of more external physical dynamics and the degree of domination by any physical symptoms of day-to-day life. The lower aspect of the transverse parameter gives the physical proportions. The upper part represents the mental aspects and is most easily assessed as the degree of intrusion or emergence of fear and anxiety symptoms into day-to-day life. These points should be assessed

separately on a 10-point scale and their combined average gives the second 'symptom'
point 0 on the graph as in Diagram 2, which is
more changeable and mobile than the first
Constitutional point.

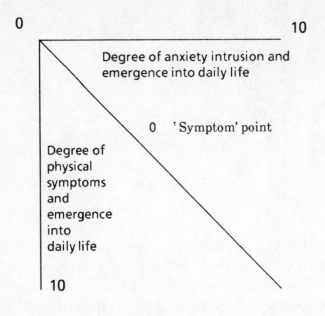

Diagram 2

The relationship between points X and 0 now
directly links the overall changeable external
expressed symptoms of the patient and their
degree of impact, intrusion, domination into
everyday life with the deeper background or
'terrain', more fixed constitutional aspects.
Both points should then be joined together and

this is best done by an elliptical curve as in Diagram 3

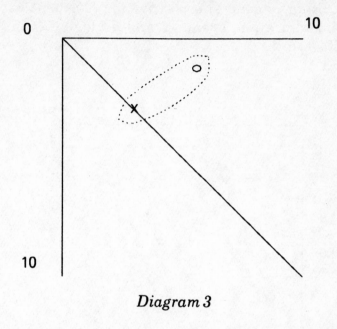

Diagram 3

Progress or otherwise by the patient can now be simply plotted from the first consultation onwards.

Examples Of Changes And Possible Use Of The Grid:

A. There is a swing upwards and outwards indicating in general a positive improvement in communication, openness and dialogue as in Diagram 4.

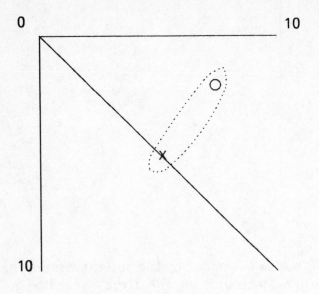

Diagram 4

B. A swing downwards and outwards indicates in general a positive change in physical constitutional energy availability and also physical well-being as Diagram 5.

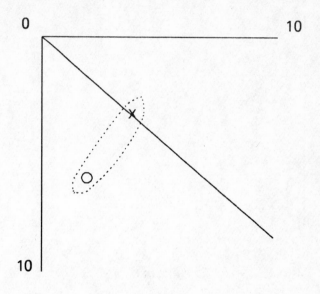

Diagram 5

C. If the swing upwards takes origin near the graph fulcrum this indicates that the domination of the patient by intrusive physical or mental symptoms is minimal as in Diagram 6.

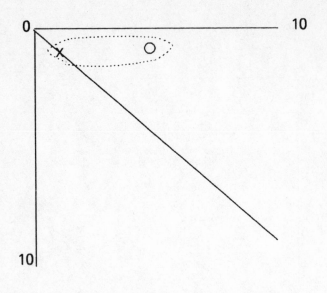

Diagram 6

D. Where the swing upwards begins more remote from the graph's fulcrum — Diagram 7, this indicates that although there is an improvement psychologically with an upwards swing, that in terms of symptoms, the patient is no better and still dominated by them at a physical or mental level or both.

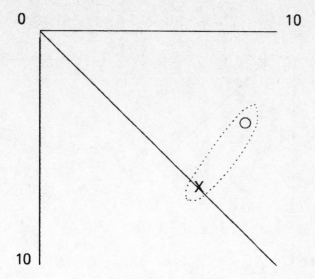

Diagram 7

E. Where the swing downwards begins remote from the fulcrum this indicates an improvement physically but that the patient is not generally better and still dominated by symptoms at a physical or mental level or both — Diagram 8.

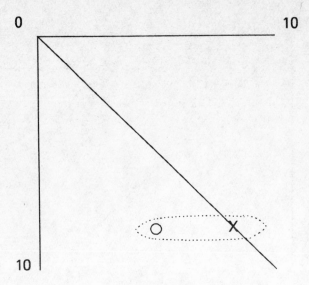

Diagram 8

Such movements give an overall indication of patient-progress and response to treatment. Changes in movements and swings can be incorporated into the grid whenever the patient is seen provided that they are allocated different colours and dated.

In this way the clinical grid gives shape and measure to clinical changes within the overall constitutional backcloth, symptom-formation and the degree, intrusion and domination by symptoms into everyday life, to lessen and limit it.

The clinical grid is a convenient way for the physician in the consulting room to measure change and movement in the most significant areas of the patient and is intended both as a research tool as well as a measure for clinical work when prescribing. The actual choice of remedy is not determined by the grid but it helps to clarify just when a change of remedy or potency is indicated.

Chapter twenty-four

Temperament

The outward expression of basic inner psychological attitudes.

Webster defines temperament as 'Man's habitual inclination, frame of mind or mode of emotional response'. It is generally what most consistently characterises personal drives, aims, motivations, energy patterns and the overall unique sense of being and relating. The inorganic, psychological expression of constitution is hung upon the more organic, less variable more solid physical constitutional frame. Temperament is the deeper psychological thread which together with the more superficial emotional responses weaves together the totality of our mentals. It gives the internal dynamo or directional force to the individual unconscious and conscious motivations, stimulating as they point the direction. Temperament fires the motor into activity, fueling ambition, need and feelings. There are sometimes strong hereditary links, and anxiety, jealousy, intolerance, insecurity, poor controls can sometimes be clearly seen as problems and weakness in other members of the family.

Chapter twenty-five

Vital Energy

The expression of the intrinsic life-force within the tissues and organ-channels maintaining health and vitality for as long as life exists. It forms and gives external shape to every impulse and energy interchange. Psychologically it manifests as awareness and impulses towards another. At organic physical depths it is responsible for the movement and production of energy at cellular levels and the processes of excretion and neurological response. Vital energy must flow uninterruptedly otherwise symptoms develop of reaction and blockage.

Note that homoeopathy cannot provide either the 'dialogue' or the specific reactions at cellular level, these are programmed at chromosomal levels, but it can provide the key-stimulus needed to start healthy movement and flow again into areas of limitation, lack or blockage. Homoeopathy can act to open gates and initiate movements of energy when lacking, or when impulses have become blocked by suppression, toxicity, physical factors and psychological damage. It is always less effective where the blockage to flow is mechanical and here a conventional approach may be initially needed so that vital energy can flow again.

Chapter twenty-six

Prognosis and Prediction in Homoeopathy

Outcome and prediction of illness depend upon a variety of differing factors all of which are important and need assessment. Most relevant are the reserves and amount of free vital-energy available and although largely inherited and constitutional, it is nevertheless markedly lessened by psychological factors as chronic stress. Other factors to be considered are the health of the 'soil' or constitutional back-ground of the patient. When this is sound and healthy, then vitality is usually good and there is an optimum degree of resilience and response by the patient.

Psychological health has a direct bearing on general health and the degree of fear, depression, withdrawal, drive and motivation is related to outcome and prognosis. The virulence and toxicity of an invading system, its resistance, motility, ability to penetrate, paralyse, speed of division, growth and spread are as important as the particular strain. Where an illness is part of an epidemic condition, toxicity may be greater than when it is an isolated occurrence. All of these are important and relevant to the presence and level of vital response by the patient and which remedy or homoeopathic potency should be given. When nutrition is poor, the person depressed, lonely or isolated without family or background support, then prognosis is different from illness in a well-nourished, healthy, optimistic temperament living within a family to give physical and psychological support.

Positive Prognostic Signs

1 A marked, short-lived (12-24 hour) aggravation or change of pattern in response to the remedy followed by an improvement.

2 The presence of a change in the intensity of symptoms or some movement within them followed by a general feeling of improvement.

3 A general sense of increased well-being by the patient although the symptoms themselves may not initially be very different.

4 The release and expression of earlier, previously repressed symptoms from the past, the patient's overall general vitality remaining high.

137

Negative Prognostic Signs:

1 The absence of any aggravation or change by the patient.

2 The patient is worse and weakening

3 The emergence of new symptoms unrelated to the past or original complaint and of a deeper more severe type.

4 There is a steady worsening of the original complaint without any true aggravation.

5 There is no general overall sense of improvement in well-being by the patient.

Psychological Prognostic Signs:

Positive

1 There is an increase in mental alertness.

2 Confidence, relaxation, openness, ease of sharing and expression is increased.

3 There is lessening of involvement with self and more caring interest and awareness of others.

Negative

1 The patient is increasingly withdrawn, frightened, deluded, remote, more preoccupied with self, illness, convictions, certainties and pessimism.

Physical Prognostic Signs:

Positive

1 A marked general increase in vitality, body-energy and body-strength.

2 There is a decrease of tension, swelling and excess feelings or reaction in the part or area affected. Spasm, pain and discomfort generally are diminished.

Negative

1 An increase in stasis, swelling, chill, tiredness, general self-awareness as well as concern and preoccupation within the area or part affected.

2 Local tension, pain, thickening or stiffness is greater with infection or reaction within the part causing discomfort, not part of an aggravation response or improvement.

As always in homoeopathy, prognosis and outcome of any condition or illness must be looked at in an overall way and not according to any recipe or formula. There are exceptions and contradictions to any illness or condition and a patient may change at any time. Situations and circumstances, both inner and outer, may vary and the most pessimistic case can suddenly take a turn for the better when psychological conditions improve. In a similar way the most positive improving patient can equally take a turn for the worse when there is a disappointment or any undermining of motivation with a marked reduction in determination, drive, vitality, optimism and life-force.

Chapter twenty-seven

Conclusions

A patient on a recent domicilliary visit said that my visit was a great comfort and very reassuring. I said that this was fine but really no part of the real aim of my visit. I had not come to reassure but to honestly inform and to perceive changes in her condition, to discuss these with her and then to prescribe or represcribe as necessary. Suggestion and reassurance were not the prime aim, although to some extent inseparable from every doctor's home visit and her needs for both clarification and reassurance. I also said that reassurance was only very short-lived and no real answer to what was needed. Sharing between doctor and patient with openness and a look at any fears may reassure but really it is only a part of the whole homoeopathic approach which should give a far more lasting tangible result than reassurance can ever provide.

Homoeopathy has the needs and causes of the patient as its highest aims. The underlying meaning of symptoms, and not just their immediate removal, eradication or replacement is part of this. Understanding an illness, why it has happened, the patient's own responsibility and role in its development is sometimes just as important as freedom from symptoms. The homoeopathic aim is not of taking away a symptom or illness in isolation from the person because this only covers up or loses important meaning. Without exception, every person is on an individual journey within his or her own spheres of experience. Learning, potential, self-development and evolving as a human being is continuous throughout life. Homoeopathy should help a little with this journey by creating the possibility and support for a greater self-expression and release of the self generally. In this way it prevents a constant re-occurrence of the same old circular problems, attitudes and blockages which cause chronic recurrent outer problems that inhibit essential inner growth and its expression as health, vitality and creativity.

Homoeopathy is not only about symptoms, potency and vital energy, it has further depths to it which are its concern to stimulate sensitivity and a greater expression of what some have called the personal inner deity, inner soul or creative force. Release of this inner mystical vitality-self which all the time seeks shape and form throughout life happens quite naturally once blocks to its expression have been resolved. With homoeopathy an individual can start to 'find' him or herself again as a real person — as so many patients have described to me. It is not the business of the physician to direct or interfere once this finding has been achieved, but it is his concern to see that it is there for each patient so that the released, unblocked creative vitality can take a more positive turn as well as an enhanced outer physical health. In this way homoeopathy supports the greatest possible expressions and happiness of the patient.

PART TWO

Chapter twenty-eight

Constitutional Prescribing

The concept of man having a constitution is a very ancient one which anticipated homoeopathy by many centuries, but the idea of there being a pattern of recognizable character and physical traits which have a relevance to prescribing is a relatively recent one. Such thinking was subsequent to the original thinking of Hahnemann, the founder of homoeopathy, who when battling with problems of chronic disease developed the theory of the hereditary miasms.

These miasms are the inherited 'flaws,' carrying the shadow or germ of illness — in one form or other, which has undermined the health and well-being of several generations within the family. Each miasm has an associated physical type of robustness and health — often a characteristic physique. The major miasm was called Psora or the 'itch', and in many ways it is related to the common chronic problem of psoriasis seen increasingly in recent years, and of unknown origin.

From Hahnemann's viewpoint, the miasms slowed down and undermined the basic constitution and its activity or vitality, causing chronic illness with typical patterns of physical and mental expressions of dysfunction. The other miasms described were Sycosis and Syphilis. These also carried the blueprint of chronic disease at chromosomal level through several generations and were responsible for dysfunction of the body as a whole. They were quite clearly shown by distortion of normal constitutional configurations and chronic intermittent illness.

Such concepts are important when prescribing for chronic, long-standing illness problems, not responding to an expected remedy or treatment indicated, but of less importance in the treatment of acute disease.

Constitution is the physiological canvas on which the psychological activities of life are both painted and enacted. It is the fundamental physical frame and basis for expression of all the wishes and intentions of the individual, which are to some degree imprinted upon it, as well as being the physical carrier of the life or vitality-force and the machinery of the spiritual and psychological sides of man. Upon this constitutional canvas are painted all the expressions of health, joy, harmony, caring and loving as well as the less noble sentiments of envy, jealousy, and the symptoms of dis-ease and ill-health. Just as in art, where the type of canvas used, its age, weave and quality, together with the supporting frame and stretchers gives the clue to the age, origins and authenticity of a painting, so too in medicine, the constitutional pictures gives the clue to past health and constitutional origins. Some would say that our present constitutional picture indicates the habits and health of several previous generations. Such knowledge and background gives added deeper meaning to many specific illnesses and symptoms of the patient relating them to the past, including the inherited past. In homoeopathy, we go back to the origins of illness, and in chronic illness, this often means going back several generations when this is possible and relevant.

We are all blessed, or otherwise, with a constitution, one that reflects hereditary patterns, the environment in which we live and the quality of our diet and life-style. Where living conditions are of lowest quality, with overcrowding, inadequate light and food, even the most well-endowed constitution may eventually become ill. But in all cases, a strongly positive constitutional pattern of health gives greater 'staying power' however inadequate the surroundings. The combination of these two forces shapes the constitutional image of the person into a recognizable unit of social functioning, familiar to self, family and friends alike. Naturally this includes the mental attributes of temperament as well as the physical, in keeping with homoeopathic principles of totality of body and mind which is the key to understanding the individual. Both must always be taken into careful consideration whenever a homoeopathic prescription is considered, in order to be accurate and effective.

As humans we are all dependent upon supplies of energy for survival and life. Such energy comes from our innate hereditary sources as well as the more obvious ones as the food we eat. The availability of energy, as well as its rate of usage (metabolism), is therefore of primary concern to the body. Constitutional vitality is closely connected to body energy efficiency and metabolic-rate. It is also related to production and storage of energy reserves, which are inseparable from strength and body stamina, as well as healthy psychological functioning.

When the energy from food — our main source of heat, is burned up too quickly because the boiler setting, or metabolic-rate of the body is too high, there is loss of weight, weakness, perspiration and exhaustion. In such cases, body fat — the equivalent of the boiler's thermal insulating jacket — is melted away and burned as excessive energy. This can only lead to greater physiological inefficiency, heat loss, and chilliness with over-activity and restlessness — mental and physical.. Here the body's combustion engine has stimulated wasteful over-activity and energy release which cannot be channelled into any useful or positive body-functioning.

Such problems occur in thyroid disease, where a toxic goitre may set energy output to an excessively high level, creating too much body heat and symptoms of sweating, weight-loss and agitation. In thyroid insufficiency, the reverse happens with a slowing down generally of energy availability and production so that the individual is cold, apathetic, without drive or vitality.

An under-active thyroid tends to occur when there is lack of essential iodine in the mineral salts of the environment, so that the gland is unable to develop and function adequately, leading to obesity and impaired metabolism. Where the constitutional system is thrown out of balance for such reasons, there is a more generalized pattern of disturbance also, involving the vitality of skin, hair, digestion and the bowels as well as an altered emotional stability. All of this can be clearly seen in thyroid disorder and shows the very general overall constitutional significance of the hormonal system as well as the importance of adequate and balanced minerals in our ecological environment for normal growth and health.

The individual is a combination of his or her constitutional machinery and inter-related psychological attitudes which form the totality of individuality. When both systems are in balance they create a situation of peace, health, relaxation and well-being. When there is lack of balance between the two there is a potentially dangerous explosive situation, and severe illness may result if the physical constitution is over-loaded with excessive emotional under-currents.

Similarly, if the body channels too much through the mind with a lack of healthy physical activity, expression, and spontaneity, excessive tension and worry may accumulate as in the typical hypochondriacal preoccupations and furrowed brow of the *Lycopodium* (club moss) make-up. In such situations everything is in the head and mental in nature, with not enough expressed by the body — in sport or exercise. When this happens, there may be so much emotional excitement, fear and general mental charge, that the body can barely function adequately or appropriately.

It is of course inconceivable to consider man as functioning solely at a mechanistic level. Although the actual machinery of man is purely physical, it is only when the psychological and inspirational elements are added — with thinking, judgement, memory, appreciation, intuition and sensitivity linked to the machine — that man finally becomes homo sapiens. But, as a human being, he also loses some of the independence of the robot and can only function fully and completely in an inter-dependent relationship, needing others for survival and fulfilment, paying the price of human vulnerability for such higher development.

The organic constitutional matrix remains constant and characteristic throughout life once adulthood has been attained. It expresses all the character, temperament and psychological attributes as well as trends in physical functioning and well-being. This totality of individual in a state of healthy equilibrium, acts as a distributor of the body's vital defences against illness. Only when the body is rigid, wooden, rock-solid in emotional attitudes and also physical functioning, does the defensive system fail to function. The bowels may then become constipated, digestion sluggish, breathing laboured and urine slow to flow. In such states, the mind is often without an original thought or feeling of significance. At such times the body is without stamina, reserve or flexibility and far more prone to disease and invasion by any one of the many viruses or bacteria present in the atmosphere.

However hygienic and clean our environment, we are all surrounded constantly by potential sources of infection and illness. Usually we are not affected by these environmental hazards because our natural constitutional resistance is high and in healthy harmony. Such constitutional vitality is under the direct influence of the mental processes and emotions, keeping the defensive patterns strong and the would-be invaders at bay. At its peak, such healthy organization radiates an obvious glow of positive health and well-being, with a spring to the step and a smile on the face. The basic overall constitution has not changed, but is in healthy balance, and this is what is needed to remain healthy and illness-free.

It is well known that when we develop a cold or infection it is nearly always because constitutional health has been previously undermined by some form of stress or strain. It is unusual for a person to develop an infection without a preceeding psychological shock or strain of some kind playing a key role in precipitating the sickness, unless physical exposure has been overwhelming or excessive in some way. Certainly, under experimental conditions, it is not sufficient just to expose the individual constitution to large dosages of the common cold virus, or to dampen and chill the extremities. In many of these cases the volunteers remain frustratingly healthy and cheerful with no sign of a cough or sneeze developing. When a constitutional pattern of natural resistance has not been undermined by trauma, shock or undue stress, there is far less susceptibility to all the common infective conditions which fill the doctor's surgery, particularly during winter months.

A healthy constitution is one full of contrasts. It has been said that inside every thin man there is a fat one struggling to get out, and within every fat person a thin one. The implication here is of an external *persona* or mask-like presentation to the world, with only a part shown externally. This is common in the smiling depressions when the tears and the desolation are kept for private expression.

Similarly with manic states — laughter and smiles are all too often a passing phase, although the true feelings of underlying defeat, devastation and sadness eventually show themselves. Temperament with all its contrasts is an inseparable part of constitution and basic attitudes, drives, psychological stamina and strengths are closely knitted to the physical. Constitution is what we are born with — our chromosomal inheritance — and this heritage interacts constantly with every aspect of our daily lives.

Energy and vitality are not just related to the amount and quality of food consumed, although this is, of course, important. Much more it relates to the level of healthy integration and balanced functioning of all the physiological parts. For some people, the amount of energy availability is such that they can only be satisfied by an overwhelming need for activity or exercise. They just cannot stay still, rest or relax, always needing to be 'on the go'.

This is characteristic for the type of temperament where the remedy *Arsenicum* may be indicated at a constitutional level provided that other physical characteristic traits are also present. Others, whatever they do and however well they feel, must sit still and relax, recovering their strength. At the least show of activity or effort they have a 'low' and feel 'all in'. For these temperaments, *Kali. carb.* may be indicated constitutionally to re-establish a better distribution of energy and build-up of reserve, helping the body to retain them and overcome feelings of depletion and chronic exhaustion.

All these variations are nothing more than the homoeopathic modalities — patterns of possible differences of the individual — the 'likes and dislikes' as recorded in the homoeopathic Materia Medica. These modality-variations give confirmatory clues to accurate prescribing and selection of the remedy, invariably reflecting the specifics of constitution and degree of healthy functioning and balance. The type of food we like — a craving for chocolate, spicy foods, or the sometimes bizarre needs of pregnancy are just one aspect of the functioning of constitution. Because such cravings take a physical form, it does not necessarily preclude underlying psychological levels of need. The craving for chocolate may relate to the need for sugar and physical energy, but equally it may be a psychological one for warmth and affection.

Chapter twenty-nine

The Body's Internal System

Constitution is the inherited arrangement of our physiological and psychological parts. At all times healthy functioning is dependent on the quality and supply of essential energy-giving nutrients as well as oxygen. The way food is presented, how it is eaten or taken in and at what speed is also relevant to energy release. But in all cases nutritional quality is fundamental. A quick snack of 'convenience', packaged food eaten at speed — just to fill a gap, only supplies the very immediate basic needs of physiological functioning. But a meal that is well-presented, lovingly prepared, eaten slowly with thought, appreciation and some reverence feeds the higher psychological spheres of man's being as well as the organic ones. It also stimulates the spiritual core of constitution which is man's very highest level of ideals and one which can integrate and harmonize both emotional and physical components of the constitutional totality.

Healthy lung functioning is a prime part of constitutional health and well-being. It is concerned with the availability and distribution of oxygen — a necessity for our fuel system in order to burn the calorie-containing food substances and release their inherent solar energy. The brain and heart are particularly vulnerable areas of energy-need with minimal reserves, and it is vital that a constant supply of oxygen be provided for their continued healthy functioning.

Similarly the heart and circulation are the pump and channels for the overall distribution of oxygen and food as potential energy and for dealing with the waste-products from the metabolic cycle within the cells. A healthy pump is essential for this constant work, and strength and efficiency can be clearly seen to be lacking where it is weak or over-laden, or there is a problem of raised blood-pressure. In such constitutions there is failure to maintain a healthy balance between heart and kidney-functioning, so that the amount of fluid in the circulation becomes excessive and cannot be eliminated. In this way the tissues become waterlogged so that breathlessness from reduced lung functioning, or swelling of the ankles occurs.

The important floral remedy *Pulsatilla* has strong action on this type of water-logged constitution, with lack of thirst a diagnostic feature, as the body fears adding the least drop of additional liquid in any form to an already saturated organism. Other relevant remedies include *Natrum mur* and *Natrum sulph.* Such severe problems within the vital physiological distributing system cause lack of energy and exhaustion. The frequently tearful disposition of the *Pulsatilla* type can be seen as a desperate bid by the body to get rid of fluid by any channel – and in such constitutions it is common to cry at the least trifle.

The digestive component of constitution varies enormously, both with efficiency, and ease of functioning and day to day needs according to energy output. It is concerned with the break-down of the energy-suppliers — foods taken in, and the elimination of indigestible, unwanted waste end-products into the stool. The function basically is to break down energy-containing food-units into simpler ones, more available to the cells as required, or used for storage pur-poses as energy reserves. This is basic and fundamental to all of us, whatever the under-lying individual constitutional organization. When digestion is interfered with for whatever reason, there may be loss of appetite, with no desire or urge to eat, so that instead of a meal being a pleasurable experience with an anti-cipatory flow of enzymic juices, there is dis-interest, pain, perhaps constipation, nausea and depression.

In some cases, the vital healthy intestinal working bacterial flora — part of the digestive back-up team, may have been killed-off or sterilized by a prolonged or excessively strong course of antibiotics leading to depleted *B*-vitamin levels, with watery diarrhoea lasting in some cases for several weeks. The exhaustion and malaise is often more a complication of treatment than a result of the original illness and it may take many weeks before these essential and normal intestinal organisms can again re-establish themselves, and digestion gets back to normal working. On the other hand, from a variety of reasons, the disturbance may have been due to a very acute infection, with inflammation of the stomach or colon. In such cases, the antibiotics may have been totally justified and necessary to treat a severe condition when no alternative therapy, such as homoeopathy, was either available, known about, or appropriate.

The kidneys are another vital aspect of constitution and include both bladder and urethra within their sphere. This renal system is absolutely vital as we are totally dependent upon its healthy functioning for the elimination of toxic wastes, that would otherwise accumulate and become fatal. Whenever vital energy is made available by combustion within the cells — inevitably waste products are produced which must be cleared from the body's energy reactor surfaces for continued health and efficient functioning. When the kidneys are working well we are blissfully unaware of their presence and functioning and it is only when there is blockage and failure that illness occurs due to the accumulation of toxins and water retention. Where the kidneys are constitionally weak for any reason, such problems are present to a lesser degree throughout life and water retention or toxic elimination may become a chronic problem, undermining health.

It is not uncommon to see successive generations of a family stricken with such chronic renal problems. An older member of the family may have had surgery for cancer of the bladder, another a chronic prostatic problem, with problems of urine flow and elimination and a younger member of the same family may have a tendency to chronic cystitis and pyelitis. Such problems often fit into the constitutional picture of remedies as *Calcarea, Natrum mur.* or *Lycopodium*, the appropriate remedy being curative, when given correctly and accurately.

The liver is the great storage organ of energy reserves for our constitution and is vital to life. Feeling 'liverish' or jaundiced is a common problem for some temperaments and a common cause of irritability. Particularly the *Nux vomica* make-up has this tendency, as also the closely related *Chelidonium* type of constitution. Healthy liver functioning is undermined by various poisons including the social ones like alcohol, tobacco or from viral disease. In some constitutions it has always been weak, inefficient, leading to a yellowish discoloration of the skin, a thin build and rapid exhaustion. Energy reserves are never good and tolerance of fats is almost nil. The liver may have been damaged earlier by an attack of hepatitis, or from occupationed toxic causes so that there is weakness due to disease as well as the constitutional limiting-factors. Healthy liver functioning is inseparable from gall-bladder efficiency so that problems of gall-stones or gall-stone colic may commonly be associated. The floral remedy *Pulsatilla* stimulates healthy liver and gall-bladder functioning and may be one of the remedies that is the key to unlocking a chronic condition of indigestion, obesity, gall-stones and misery going back over many years. But there are other equally important hom-oeopathic remedies that would also need to be considered before a final choice of remedy was decided upon.

When we look at the variations possible in the circulation it is found that these vary enormously. Some at the first sign of winter develop chilblains and are always chilly, as is typical of the rather fussy *Arsenicum* make-up. Others seem always too hot, and rarely wear a coat on the coldest day — indicating perhaps a *Sulphur* constitution. Yet others have a constant tendency to varicose veins, the limbs blue with swollen ankles and heavy, lead-like legs. Such a poor circulation may be an additional feature that indicates *Pulsatilla* or *Lachesis* as their constitutional prescription. The *Pulsatilla* make-up is chilly on the warmest day as well as totally intolerant of heat in any form, so that it is the remedy par excellence for paradox and variability. In others the skin feels cold, sweaty and limp, totally lacking in tone and vigour, indicating *Calcarea* as a possible remedy of choice.

Whatever the varieties and variations of the constitutional make-up, each individual is inevitably different and no two are exactly alike — even identical twins — and homoeopathy makes no attempt to contradict this or to impose a rigid system of classification or treatment in order to type-cast patients, which would be totally alien to all homoeopathic traditions. Constitution is the background cloth, giving the setting to the particular period of life but given its characteristic impetus by the aims, mental needs and psychological drives of the time. These 'call the tune', the stage is the inherited constitution which has to be used to its best possible advantage. The notion of constitutional types is of undoubted value in giving the clue to the type of functioning, background and physiology of the individual so that a remedy can be matched with the physical configurations, and a potency adapted to the degree of involvement of psychological elements in the symptoms, giving accuracy and depth when prescribing.

Classification of Constitutions

If we look at some of the earlier attempts to understand constitutional prescribing, we find that many of the earlier homoeopaths classified according to homoeopathic remedies, and in many ways in the best traditions of homoeopathic thinking and understanding of the patient.

Clarke in his *Dictionary of Domestic Medicine* described three basic constitutional types:

Calcarea, with clammy hands and chilly irritability;

Sulphur, which is hot and perspiring, with an irritable skin and a faint sinking sensation in the stomach with typical left-sided problems;

Lycopodium, where flatulence, constipation and right-sided problems predominate.

Grauvogl's Classification

In *Constitutional Medicine* Clarke discusses the Grauvogl concepts of constitution in detail and deals with his three major divisions of physical types as follows:

The Hydrogenoid Constitution

Here there is an excess of water and fluid in the tissues which corresponds to Hahnemann's Sycosis classification type and the major remedy *Thuja*.

The Oxygenoid Constitution

In this type of make-up there is an excess of oxygen present in the tissues which leads to a burning up and break-down of both nutrition and tissue cells. This corresponds well with

Hahnemann's original classification group of Syphilis and the major indicated remedies — *Mercurius* and *Kali iodatum*.

The Carbo-Nitrogenoid Constitution.

Nutrition of all tissues is slowed down and retarded to a marked degree with lethargy and exhaustion prime symptoms because of insufficient oxygen to the body's essential organs and tissues. It corresponds to Hahnemann's major miasmic grouping of Psora. Major associated remedies are *Sulphur, Argentum nitricum, Nux vomica* and *Natrum sulph.*

Guernsey's Classification

Writing in *Homoeopathic Domestic Principles* Guernsey describes the following physical constitutional types for consideration by the homoeopathic practitioner.

Plethoric	Robust, high blood-pressure type of make-up.
Feeble	Lacking in strength, animal heat and warmth and energy.
Bilious	Where liver and gall-bladder are weak, the skin yellowish.
Apoplectic	Thick-set and impulsive, pulse and blood-pressure variable.

Nervous	Over-sensitive and excitable, the temperament weak and changeable.
Lymphatic	Sluggish, weak and catarrhal with a tendency to water-retention.
Catarrhal	With general lack of vitality, particularly of the skin.
Consumptive	The individual is pale and tall with tendencies to chest weakness.

Vannier's Classification

The eminent French homoeopath emphasised in all his writings the importance of the following constitutional patterns of posture and temperament. He described the following groups:

Carbonic

There is rigidity and stiffness of the whole body as well as of mental attitudes. Both upper and lower limbs tend to be held permanently in a position of partial flexion with the body slightly bent forwards all the time. Rhythmic order, reliability and responsibility are marked in the temperamental attitudes. This type of make-up is often helped by *Calcarea carbonica*.

Phosphorus

Here the patient tends to be more tall and thin and often rather elegant. Arms and legs are held perfectly straight at all times and there is a rather distinctive grace and supple quality to every movement. In temperament they are a mixture of the artistic and perfectionism. Their remedy is often *Phosphorus*.

Fluoric

In direct contrast to the Carbonic make-up the Fluoric posture is one of the limbs being fixed in a position of extension and rather bent backwards which causes the typical irregularity and instability of their posture and movement. They are nearly always uncoordinated in some way, 'double-jointed' with a temperament which is both accident-prone and 'out of true' like the limb positioning and needing considerable help and guidance from others. *Calcarea fluorica* is usually their indicated remedy.

All these groupings and classifications have their intrinsic advantages as well as disadvantages, particularly the latter when considering the uniqueness of the individual. Their merit is of pointing out the various possibilities of physiological functioning and its relevance to prescribing. Any stimulus to looking at the person as an individual has value, and we are all inevitably part of some group, albeit a social one. Provided that such classifications are carefully looked at as pointers and a stimulus to thought only, they are helpful. Their danger is of being a pigeon-hole to either the patient or the prescriber.

My own personal preference and as an aid only to prescribing in the constitutional maze is to consider the following groups of related physical characteristics when working out the constitutional prescription.

Obese-phlegmatic

Where slowness and passivity are marked with lack of muscular strength and drive and a general tendency to hold-back both physically and mentally. (*Calcarea*)

Thin-impulsive

Here in contrast, quickness and impulsiveness are the rule with impatience at both physical and psychological levels. Everything is done too quickly and this may in part account for the failure to retain either body fat or fluids as well as ideas. (*Arsenicum*)

Disorganised-unrealistic

Untidyness, remoteness and unreality is common as much physically as emotionally and close bodily contact is usually avoided although at the same time dependence and passivity may also be marked. Everything is put off, delayed or fobbed-off in some way so that experience and confidence is never truly built-up. (*Sulphur*)

Fearful-restless

Here the body is dominated by an over-anxious fearful temperament which affects the whole of body functioning from a weak digestive system with indigestion and flatulence to weak bowels with diarrboea or the heart with palpitations. Anticipation, conviction and negative certainty are so strong that the whole of constitutional healthy functioning is undermined by it. (*Lycopodium*)

The Commoner Remedies For Each Group:

Obese-phlegmatic

Warm- blooded   *Pulsatilla, Kali carb.*

Cold- blooded   *Calcarea*

Thin-impulsive

Warm- blooded   *Phosphorus*

Cold- blooded   *Nux vomica, Medorr-*
                       hinum, Arsenicum

Disorganised-unrealistic

Warm- blooded   *Sulphur Natrum mur*

Cold- blooded   *Silicea*

Fearful-restless

Warm- blooded   *Aconitum, Argentum*
                       nitricum. Belladonna
Cold- blooded   *Lycopodium*

Illness may be considered as a reaction to environmental stress due to the emotional pressures of our modern jet-age society, inevitably creating frustration and tension because everything now has to be done and adjusted to in a *minimum* of time. All too often there is impatience and lack of faith or conviction in whatever is being done. These environmental strains inevitably fall upon the organic constitution via the emotions, draining resistance and body reserves. They add to any inherited miasmic flaws already present in a particular organ or physiological system — the liver perhaps, or circulatory organs.

Such dual pressures create rigidity and a 'locked up', more vulnerable state with impatience, anxiety and an increased disposition to such everyday illnesses as 'flu', the common cold and viral infections generally. There is loss of normal constitutional tone in the underlying organs and their associated physiological systems become out of tune, leading to jaded, exhausted feelings. This is clearly shown in the scalp and hair which tends to become lifeless and drab without its usual bounce. The skin may also lack vitality and be more prone to acne. Often the fingers become swollen, or there may be extreme fatigue, particularly in a young person. In general there is no recognizable illness present at first, but the individual is below par, without reserves of energy. If activity is continued at the same high level with the same stresses and environmental strains, a more definable and recognizable illness must eventually set in as the condition worsens and the pressures increase.

Chapter thirty

Threats to Constitutional Health

The homoeopathic prescription aims to treat and resolve any early situation where constitutional health is undermined. Major factors which put pressure on the constitution are as follows:

Stress

This is something unfortunately with which we are all familiar and the major economic and social difficulties which we now face only serve to aggravate the already unrealistic demands made by society for accelerated pace and changes without adequate psychological preparation. Pressures in the work-field have now become a major issue, and unemployment is still at an all-time high.

Pollution

The major areas of damage are those caused by excessive vibration and noise, particularly in the urban concrete of our cities where many work in offices under artificially controlled conditions frequently with no natural light throughout the working day. Further weakening factors are the additives and preservatives present in our foods, artificially prolonging their natural keeping and storage-life to lessen waste at the expense of undermining nutritional value. The air we breathe is now heavily polluted, particularly by carbon monoxide and toxic lead wastes. So, too, is our water supply — contaminated by fluorides and chemical 'purifiers' of unknown long-term significance for health. Tobacco and alcohol are the other common social pollutants which can undermine the healthiest.

The Quality of Food

This is often below any acceptable standard, particularly the instant or fashionable convenience food and seems to relate clinically to the high degree of ill-health seen in many young people of today. This is particularly a danger in the younger school-child, where both central catering and pre-packed lunches leave much to be desired nutritionally. The adolescent is also very vulnerable to media publicity for packaged foods of nutritionally dubious quality.

Drugs

The so-called aids to health are also part of the convenience-living movement in society today. 'I have a headache, or an attack of indigestion — so I must have something to instantly get rid of it, because it is not *convenient* to have pain or discomfort'. So we have a plethora of drugs on the market — many sold over the counter for the instant relief of almost anything. There are drugs for the relief of headache, indigestion, diarrhoea, constipation, plus all the numerous vitamins and pick-me-up pills as well as the appetite-suppressants. None of these are without their risk to the healthy constitution, which is often and quite simply 'out-of-phase' temporarily — for reasons of excess, or from the generalized environmental stresses. The dangers of such drugs far exceed the risk of a headache to the system — but it is fashionable and therefore we must have it.

Lack of Exercise

This is another drain on the health of the constitution. Until recently a regular daily walk was always called a 'constitutional', and it was recognized as toning-up of the body generally. We live our lives locked-up in cars, on polluted motorways so that little remains of any natural rhythmic relationship with nature, our environment or the seasons. In general, and with minor exceptions, less and less concern is being taken of the body, and less responsibility

taken by the individual for its level of functioning and health.

As far as the mind is concerned both critical
and creative faculties are being rapidly eroded
away by the excess pressures of the media to
sell an increasingly sophisticated technology
where the quality of soft-ware and programmes
circulated lags considerably behind technical
advance. Particularly television is responsible
for much of the current passivity and lack of
orginality which is increasingly prevalent.

When the constitution is less flexible, we then
become more vulnerable to illness, less able to
mobilize resistance and natural immunity so
that symptoms and allergy may develop,
making us more susceptible to depression or
obesity. How common for the homoeopath to
give the constitutional remedy to a patient in
the 'high' 10M potency and to see after 48 hours
that the patient is better psychologically,
having resolved a problem or a decision that
had been worrying him or her for weeks or
months. In addition the patient has often unblocked an impasse in the bowels, or perhaps a
large strangulated torturing pile has cleared
up within a matter of hours together with an
associated depressive problem.

Sometimes the whole of the constitutional
system feels out of balance. There is water retention, swelling of the ankles, a puffy face,
headache, blood-pressure, diarrhoea or sometimes constipation. All of these physical aspects

of individual constitution are held in a state of healthy balance by the mind and its quality and degree of feelings and attitudes, so that healthy functioning of internal organs is much more than just one of endocrine control. It is also deeply psychological, and closely related to the emotional. This can be clearly seen in those problems of anxiety or stress which have an overwhelming effect on normal bowel-functioning, kidney or digestive systems, so that indigestion, peptic ulceration, nervous urinary frequency or severe colitis may occur.

Both conscious and unconscious levels of mind play a key role in balancing and supporting the health of the major physiological organs. Such a controlling link can be seen where techniques of suggestion by hypnosis are used experimentally to reverse or inhibit normal allergy or immune response on one side of the body – for example the T.B. Mantoux test. Most people now agree that the major allergies as hay fever, eczema, or asthma have clearly marked psychological triggers and that the mental attitudes and emotional tensions play as important a role in their prevention as dust and pollen levels in the atmosphere.

Obesity is a common faulty attempt by the body to compensate for constitutional insufficiency and weakness by excess eating and 'snacking'. Because the basic constitution is under pressure and out-of-equilibrium, the inherent weakness is wrongly put down to hypoglycaemia or hunger and a need for food. The additional weight further weakens health by promoting water retention and additional body fat. There is an empty, 'all gone' sensation, difficult to define with almost canine hunger — even after food. Such details can give the clue to the precise constitutional remedy needed, and one which has the power to correct the underlying imbalance and rigidity. *Sepia* or *Sulphur* might be thought of for the above symptoms. Often there is a depressive factor which further contributes to compulsive eating, but at a more superficial level than any underlying constitutional malaise and imbalance.

Excess weight always puts a strain upon the kidneys, stomach and heart. The weakened kidneys have already to cope with excreting an excessive amount of waste by-products to maintain health in balance. Fluid retention is commonly present and the very tissues themselves feel cold, damp, soggy, almost waterlogged. This is the typical picture of the constitutional make-up where *Calcarea* is indicated or sometimes *Natrum mur*.

If we now consider the individual symptoms within the context of the constitutional whole, they have at a different level of significance to the much deeper organic matrix of the physiological system. Symptoms occur artificially in the 'similar' or proving experiments when the homoeopathic remedy is repeatedly given to a group of healthy, symptom-free volunteers until a reaction or sensitivity occurs.

When considering constitutional make-up, it is the background that is observed – the sub-soil from which symptoms emerge and take root, – familial and hereditary tendencies rather than any individual symptoms which may be infinitely variable. Constitutional prescribing is concerned with this deeper organic physical state of the individual, which both binds and expresses the symptom picture. It provides the possibility for a wide variety of symptoms and complaints as is completely documented in the Materia Medica, particularly that of Kent and Boenninghausen where all possible symptom-variations are arranged in a logical order from which the remedy may be chosen.

The constitutional type gives the lead to the doctor as to the group of remedies to look for and those which may be particularly needed at some stage in the treatment, particularly in problems of chronic illness. When the constitutional make-up of the individual and the Materia Medica agree as to the symptom-remedy, then this can be confidently given in highest potency of 200c or more with positive results.

Homoeopathy is the science of individualization. Its concern is to assess the blocks which cause the unique personal potential inherent in everyone, physically as well as and psychologically, to be locked away and unrealized because of stress-provoked illness and weakness. Where natural drives and potential are unable to be channelled into creative outlets and circuits which generate ideas and express feelings and sensitivity, then a situation of frustration and chronic illness can develop. Prescribed accurately and in sufficiently high potency, the homoeopathic remedy can release this central vitality so that health is kept at an optimum. For the individual patient, the constitutional remedy can stimulate the beginning of this unlocking by a prescription that facilitates both the emergence and the freeing of the total person at physical and psychological levels.

The primary cause of all illness is an undermined and weakened constitutional organization and defensive patterns, which make the individual particularly vulnerable at its weakest link – its weakest organ which is often the entry-point for infection and disease into the vital energy system. Such an organ is usually weak from hereditary reasons, often throughout several generations, being an Achilles' heel for several members of the family. When the cause is a hereditary miasm, undermining the functioning of the organ, then the constitutional remedy can be the first step to correcting its inherent weakness, although one of the more specific nosodes or tissue-origin remedies may also be needed at a later date to complete the prescription.

In one way or another, many patients seen are 'locked up' within themselves, both physically and emotionally. The constitutional remedy can ease this 'locked' position where nothing else seems to be happening in terms of growth, health or achievement, at psychological or physical levels. The constitutional remedy can un-freeze these blockages so that the patient is also more amenable to the lower potencies, which work at a more tangible symptomatic level.

This constitutional well-being gives the patient more capacity to respond to both opportunities and environment, aided by the enhanced physical health and greater energy availability. Because we are all living under stress at some time, it is important for every patient to have a constitutional prescription at some time in order to lessen the possibility of long-standing or chronic problems developing.

For all but the most superficial tissue-level type of problem, constitutional therapy is essential as the stresses and strains of modern living have become so widespread and generalised. This is especially true in urban life where pressures are far greater. Even those actively involved with an exciting creative job are still under pressure and no longer immune from stress. They often need to prove and to justify themselves, creating and engendering more pressure and work at a time of maximum demand. This can make them illness-prone and at their peak of youth and output, they are often ill with recurrent catarrh, colds or allergy problems. When this occurs it is often only the constitutional remedy that effects a real and permanent cure.

The polycrests or remedies of multiple broad-range action are the major constitutional remedies, as they have an influence on every major system of the body, creating balance, resilience and health. There should be no confining of homoeopathic prescribing to the limits of these polycrest remedies however and every well-prescribed appropriate constitutional remedy is able to unblock both mental attitudes and physical aspects when all else has failed.

It facilitates greater and more accurate perception and judgement, so that the patient gradually becomes more accessible, less rigid and caught-up in his or her situation. As a result of this type of approach, problems previously seen as insoluble, and perceived from one particular viewpoint, are able to be seen in a better and fuller light and with perspective.The freeing of psychological perspectives as well as physical well-being gives the greatest possibility for maximum health, insight and well-being.

Chapter thirty-one

Constitutional Prescribing and Cancer

In conclusion to this section, I would like to make some comments on the relevance of homoeopathic constitutional prescribing to cancer formation and its prevention. The paragraphs which follow make no claim whatsoever that homoeopathy can cure cancer or even that it has a major part to play in established disease of this type. I do feel, however, that the constitutional approach may have an important role to play in prevention. Such thoughts are at best purely personal and individual, and might even be called 'speculative'.

Nevertheless, I do feel that they are sufficiently important to be shared, as long as it is appreciated that what follows does not in any way constitute a definitive statement as to cancer formation or its cure by homoeopathic methods. My interest and concern is one of research into prevention and the possible role of the homoeopathic constitutional prescription in this field. The reasons for stating my present position and thinking at a relatively early stage is the hope of sharing and stimulating ideas and thought-links – perhaps feed-back from others – either present patients, or former ones as well as from other workers in this field.

Following discussion with adult cancer patients and their families over the years who have made successful recoveries, taking into account their purely subjective viewpoints and opinions as to possible causes and related factors that may have triggered-off the disease, I have come to the following working hypothesis as to some of the major causative elements. I am deliberately excluding from these present ideas the terrible problem of cancer in children as it seems to be of a different order, with a much more rapid and severe dis-organisation than in the adult illness.

In all the cases discussed, I have been struck by the undeniable common patterns that emerge in most cases, both in men or women, which is that there has been a previous often sudden and severe stress or pressure occurring in the previous six to twelve months before the onset of the cancer process but which did not lead to the development of any other apparent external illness or disease at the time.

Typical causative stress factors described are a sudden loss, tragedy, illness or incapacity in a close member of the family. Often they have had to support and nurse them as patients over a period of several weeks or months at the expense of their own reserves.

In others, the shock has been at a more individual, private, personal level with no exhausting person to suffer, carry and care for. But in nearly all cases the shock and stress has been severe and obvious to those closest and most involved with the individual concerned. Especially, and most important of all, there tends to be no outward declaration, or sharing of the emotional pressures. In keeping with their general pattern and temperament, they stoicly put up and get on with it — whatever the cost to themselves.

Personal guilt feelings are also commonly associated with the emotional stress or pressures. In every case the pressures were buried — often deeply, in keeping with the tendency to keep everything — physically and emotionally, unexpressed, suppressed and denied. Over the years they have always done this, reflecting unhealthy psychological patterns that are too intense, being over-conscientious, often proud, hard-working, perfectionistic and self-sacrificing to a fault. They are the load-bearers of the family. Because of their marked sense of responsibility they easily become life's scapegoats, always uncomplaining. Although not lacking in anger and resentment, such feelings are only rarely shown and then only in a moderated, controlled degree. In general however they are neither voiced nor made obvious or admitted to.

This type of personality make-up does not usually develop recognizable forms of psychological illness or outlet-symptoms whatever the degree of pressure, stress or strain so that there is no tendency to form a depressive or anxiety illness as might be expected, given the circumstances. Nor is there a marked phase of 'irritable' complaints like indigestion, insomnia, backache, exhaustion or collapse. In fact a doctor is rarely needed because they are rarely ill until the cancer change occurs. All feeling, associated emotions and reactions are consistently denied, suppressed and buried, what-ever the demand or circumstance. Usually there is no common psychosomatic manifestation either from the pressures as asthma, eczema, diabetes or rheumatoid arthritis, which might be expected and understandable. Similarly the other more severe physical expressions of blocked emotion as colitis are rare. Only headaches, constipation, a faded appetite are common, with eventual total loss of interest in food.

Such psychosomatic illnesses seem to serve a fundamental protective outlet function for the body amongst other things, particularly as far as cancer is concerned, and when they fail to occur with all reactions and feelings pushed down to the deepest possible levels, this allows no alternative pathway of exit for the body to react with. This unhealthy, undesirable position is a reflection of the degree which suppressant tendencies within the personality can affect, overwhelm and even devastate physical health. In this way all the superficial and deeper pathways of outlet both physical and psychological are kept closed so that the mental reactions of fatigue and stress are retained at their deepest and most dangerous level of the constitution − where it is most vulnerable − namely at levels of vital organ and cellular regeneration functioning.

Under such circumstances, the patterns of normal constitutional resistance are slowly lowered so that fatigue and exhaustion are felt at an early stage, although appetite and bowel disturbance − usually in the form of a reduced appetite and constipation occur soon afterwards.

In general other members of the family are invariably well looked after, often with great caring and typical dedication but at a considerable price because of masochism and self-sacrifice.

Case Report I

A women of 57 came with breast cancer. There was a history of a similar condition in the colon 25 years earlier, treated surgically at that time. She quite clearly stated that the condition had been brought on by stress from shortage of money over several years. She had felt drained of all energy, and became anaemic. For several months before the cancer became apparent, she had worked excessively hard without a proper break, with lots of young people in the home, becoming 'low' and too tired to eat or nourish herself properly. She had lived mainly on milky tea, biscuits and cake, although preparing balanced meals for the rest of the family. In this way she severely crippled her own constitution, denying it all the essential vitamins with a diet which was abnormally high in refined starches plus the inevitable preservatives, additives and colourants that are now part of every shop-bought confectionery. One day she felt something 'snap' in her and irreversibly 'changed'. Cancer developed some six months later.

Case Report II

A woman of 40 came after a gap in consultations of 6 years. When last seen she was tearful and depressed because of the break-up of her marriage but otherwise well. Examination showed two separate cancerous growths in the same breast. She stated that the growths had begun at a time of stress following the breakdown of a four-year relationship which had ended a year previously. She described 'the process of her divorce, moving to a new flat, and changing offices at work'. After the break-up she felt hurt, under great strain, that he had 'made a fool of her'. She spent most of her day crying because of the hurt. He had recently married and she felt that her man had been stolen from her, but — "he won't have my breast as well !". She got to a stage when she could not be alone, could only sit crying, unable to cope — with dreams of being lost in a strange town and forgetting where she had left her car. All of this reflected her severe state of psychological confusion.

Others live on excesses of coffee or cigarettes — both highly suspect cancer factors. Some, still, indulge in equally harmful excessive spicy or sweet foods, craving particularly chocolate, which is taken instead of a more balanced diet and as an alternative and compensation for the abnormally and deeply displaced stress problems. Like all suppressed diseases, such problems are far more difficult for the body to cope with and its defensive machinery to deal with, once it is buried so deeply as to be less available for the normal adjustment and compensation to take place.

In recent papers (1975 and 1978). Greer describes similar work with cancer patients at the Department of Psychological Medicine, King's College Hospital. The main psychological factors in the activity of cancer were related to a rigid conforming temperament, with self-criticism marked, depression and stress. In many cases there were problems of deep anxiety, deferred hope, denial and repression together with hopelessness and disappointment.

Such deep-seated feelings are usually directly linked to either the hormonal or cortico-steroid immune-system pathways through the mid-brain, but especially with the hypothalamus. These would seem to play a major role in tumour development.

Greer studied 160 women under 50 years old admitted to King's for biopsy with breast lumps of unknown type. Of the women, 69 were found to have cancerous growths; the rest were benign. There was a clearly positive correlation between the group of women with cancer and the patterns of suppressed rage and anger. Abnormal serum-immunoglobulin IgA levels were correlated to the women with suppressed anger in both the benign as well as the cancerous groups.

As Greer comments, statistical correlation does not mean anything other than this and a definite cancer link cannot be concluded from the figures. But it is highly suggestive that suppression of anger, abnormal serum-immunoglobulin levels and cancer may be linked. It also confirms the clinical observations of many physicians, including my own experience.

The combination of lowered constitutional resistance, fatigue, a diet deficient in essential vitamins — improverished in quality, together with deeply denied and suppressed psychological pressures and resentment or guilt can severely undermine the normal patterns of body vitality. When potentially cancer-forming agents are liberally taken in addition and to excess, then this combination is sufficient in some cases to provoke abnormal patterns of cellular growth which can then organise themselves into new growth spirals with their own particular pattern of rules and proliferation. In this way a new cellular nucleus develops, immune to the usual patterns of defence, partly because they are not functioning adequately and sufficiently to be able to inhibit such growths at an early stage while they are still controllable.

All of us are normally protected from these new growth centres developing by a combination of hereditary vitality, hormonal balance and cancer 'antibodies' in our constitutional make-up. There fundamental factors prevent and destroy abnormal cellular formations as they occur. But given the above physical and psychological conditions, the constitutional cancer-protective forces are undermined. Such forces are in many ways like a positive hereditary miasm. Earlier we looked at miasms in a purely negative light — as a 'flaw' and as carriers of disease patterns and tendencies into the constitution. But there are also the more positive constitutional inherited factors too which strongly protect the healthy organization. It is these 'defensive' miasmic factors which permit some constitutions to drink and smoke excessively, often into old age — with a diet that is nutritionally doubtful, yet remaining apparently youthful and with no familial or individual tendency to new growth formation.

Whilst in no way talking of a homoeopathic cure for cancer, I believe that the best approach should be one of prevention whenever possible. The individual constitutional remedy, given in a sufficiently high potency of 200c or more, can mobilise and stimulate constitutional reorganization back into a more healthy position where positive anti-cancer factors, normally present in health are free to act again. Any severe nutritional deficiency must also be corrected at the same time and obvious psychological knots allowed to emerge and unravel. The individual constitutional has the power to untangle many suppressed psychological problems so that they can be more easily dealt with by the normal patterns and procedures of psychological functioning and defence without the dangers that radical suppression and burial-in-depth brings.

In a situation where there is a family history of cancer, the normal inherited protective miasmic factors weak, or when an overwhelming shock or pressure has occurred or been denied, together with vitamin and constitutional impoverishment, I suggest that the individual constitutional remedy be given. The reason it is indicated is because of its important positive and protective role to health.

If we are ever to begin to deal with this scourge of our present society it is important that treatment is not just concerned with an approach *after* the event — important though this is. It is just as important, if not more so, to approach the problem prophylactically by prevention, especially in those known to be especially vulnerable. As well as developing advanced techniques in surgery, radioactive and x-ray treatment, chemotherapy and diagnosis, we must also try to inhibit abnormal cell formation at its source and origin.

In this way the classical homoeopathic approach and concepts of constitutional prescribing may work side by side with modern and sophisticated medical techniques. Helping patients to bring patterns of denial or suppression to the surface by a safe remedy that both releases and mobilises the natural individual vital defences may be of inestimable value. But more research is needed and these comments are only by way of an approach to a difficult problem. Let us not forget that however exciting and important the advances in modern medicine, surgery, diagnosis and treatment — in all cases prevention is always better than cure.

Chapter thirty-two

Major Constitutional Types

The Aconitum Constitution

Mentals:

Tension with agitation, restlessness and fear is the keynote of the remedy. This is seen at a mental level with anxiety, marked fright and a fear of death; at a vascular level with haemorrhages; at the muscular level with spasm, tetanus and asthma. There is numbness – as if the body and limbs were bound tightly. They are quarrelsome, changeable, easily angered, with a marked fear of crowds and of going out, certain that they are going to die and predicting the exact time and hour when it will happen.

General Indications for Aconitum as a remedy:

One of the best, most reliable remedies for acute illnesses and inflammations of children, especially useful in the first 24 hours but no later than 48 hours. Also useful in adult acute conditions. The common cause is exposure and chill from dry cold winds. Also for fear, fright, shock and injury. Usually for lively, healthy strong, highly coloured, stout people, with dark hair.

Site of Action:

Inflammation of outer and middle ear, throat, tonsils, larynx and chest.

Symptoms:

High fever and severe, sharp, tearing, shooting, stitch-like and insuppressable pains, violent in onset. The skin is red hot and dry, although the patient feels chilled and the pulse is full and bounding. The face is flushed and swollen, cheek red, tongue swollen, coated thick white or yellow-white, itching and burning. Cough, earache, croup, asthma are all common; often bright red blood is coughed up or passed, with breathing loud and laboured. Chest is hot and tight. Facial paralysis due to chill from a cold wind.

Modalities:

Better for: Open air, rest.

Worse for: Dry cold air, noise, music, heat, touch, uncovering, evening before midnight.

The Arsenicum Constitution

Mentals:

Nervous and restless from mental anxiety, easily taking fright and fearing death. They are both irritable and miserable, easily becoming angry or depressed, often hopeless or despairing. The basic personality is rigid, fastidious, precise and fussy, over-sensitive to noise, touch, excitement, and surroundings generally. They are often fearful of being alone, or going out alone, and are generally terrified of paternal figures.

General Indications:

These are primarily of nervous restlessness, prostration with exhaustion, burning pains, and the mental picture in thin pale subjects, thirsty for little but often. The least demand causes a loss of strength.

Site of Action:

Arsenicum affects the body generally, but in particular it has strong actions upon mucous membranes of the gastro-intestinal tract and respiratory system.

Symptoms:

Arsenicum is an acute remedy, although it may be helpful in chronic disease when there is marked prostration and restlessness. They are cold, chilly people who hug the fire and radiators. Asthma is common and when acute they need to sit up to breathe, finding it impossible to lie down because of a burning, suffocating sensation. The face is often pale, puffy, drawn and haggard, which ages them. The burning pains and sensations are better for heat and hot drinks. There are many gastrointestinal symptoms — as gastric ulcer, cancer, colic and cramps — always of a burning exhausting character. Arthritis is common, with unbearable drawing burning pains and cramps in the fingers, wrists, hips, arms and hands. Frequently the ankles are puffy and swollen. Haemorrhage from the stomach, intestine or rectum is frequent. The skin is cold, pale and clammy, often itching and burning. *Arsenicum* particularly enjoys fats of all types, and feels better for rain.

Modalities:

Better for: Heat, rest, hot drinks, lying in bed with the head high,.

Worse for: Midnight until 1.00 a.m., cold, an ice cream or cold drinks, the damp, lying on the affected side with the head low.

The Bryonia Constitution

Mentals:

Irritable, restless, anxious, often concerned unneccessarily about the future. They become angry at the least thing, often difficult people, easily disturbed. At times they are very talkative but at other times there is a sluggish state of mind. They feel depressed and the head feels confused.

General Indications:

Usually they are well-built with dark complexion and hair, often the onset has been due to cold from exposure to a dry cold east wind, and usually the symptoms come on slowly.

Site of Action:

Bryonia mainly affects the mucous membrane with dryness of the mouth. lips, throat, nose, stomach and intestine, due to impaired secretions. The serous lining membranes of the chest are inflamed with pneumonia, pleurisy, or a simple cough. The abdominal organs, especially liver and kidneys are affected, and there are also haemorrhages and joint involvement.

Symptoms:

Dryness is the feature of the remedy — the lips crack, the tongue is dry and white-coated, and the mouth and throat are dry needing copious drinks of cold water, but taken infrequently to minimise any movement which always typically aggravates the *Bryonia* stitch-like pains. There is dry cough and constipation with large dry hard brown or black crumbling faeces due to the lack of intestinal secretions. The face is hot, swollen and red, and there are dry sticking pains in the sternum, or sides of the chest, often right-sided and always better for local pressure or lying on the side of the pain or inflammation. Vertigo and dizziness are a feature, usually worse in the morning on rising, as also headache — usually frontal, often right-sided, worse for bending, stooping, and in the morning.

The scalp is tender, nose bleeds are common, better for a cold compress as also the toothache which is improved by cold water. *Bryonia* patients have painful periods with lancing, stitching dysmenorrhoea, improved by cool applications. The stomach is painful when eating, heavy as if a stone is inside, and offensive flatus is passed. The breasts feel heavy, indurated, stony hard and may be pale or red, hot or inflamed, as in mastitis. The legs feel weak, weary and heavy and generally there is fainting and great exhaustion, often severe on waking. Rheumatism of knees, wrists and hands, the joints red, swollen and painful, often right-sided.

Modalities:

Better for: Local pressure, cool air, cold applications, lying on the affected side, lying quietly still, for sweating.

Worse for: Touch, movement, the least jar or pressure — covers are often kicked off. Stooping and bending aggravate — especially the headaches — heat, in the morning, the evening from 9 p.m. to midnight, sitting up, damp weather.

The Calcarea Constitution

Mentals:

Calcarea people are full of anxiety, fear and apprehension. They worry over everything and are depressed, but can usually be roused out of their states of gloom by reassurance and attention without too much difficulty. They are obstinate, wake at night about 3.00 a.m. with night terrors and generally tend to be restless, forgetful and confused — often twitching and trembling, and at times in state of complete delirium. They have disturbing dreams as of death, and generally there is a rumination and phantasy over morbid subjects.

General Indications:

The principle indications are the sense of chilliness, damp hands and feet in a rather fat, clumsy, soft and flabby, overweight, fair-haired person, lacking general body, skin and muscular tone. Growth generally is slow, the milestones delayed, such as teething, and they tend to have a larger head, with a pale skin, and display weakness, exhaustion, and a proneness to sweating.

Site of Action:

Calcarea affects the whole body, but most of all the mind, nervous system, chest, abdomen and joints.

Symptoms:

Chilly and cold, with damp hands and feet, a tendency to sweat profusely at night in bed, so that the pillow is often quite moist. Pallor, lack of tone, soft flabby tissues and body with chalky white appearance is characteristic. Sourness is a pointer to this remedy, with loss of taste and smell, so that everything smells or tastes sour, as also the stools and urine. The urine can sometime contain bright red blood. Incontinence may occur.

Lymph glands may be enlarged in the neck and groin. There are many digestive difficulties — including abnormal cravings for eggs, soap, cinders, slate, pencils, chalk and coal.

Although the appetite is considerable they are not relieved by eating and almost immediately afterwards experience a 'sinking' sensation, often present on waking. The abdomen is enlarged, and colicky pains occur. Diarrhoea is a chalky pale undigested stool with the characteristic sour odour.

Mental deficiency is sometimes associated with anaemia, tuberculosis or rickets. Together with coldness and dampness, there is also a burning which may occur in the rectum and also on the top of the head, causing profuse perspiration. The feet are often burning hot and have to be pushed out of the bed and hot flushes are a feature. The *Calcarea* patient not only flushes up easily but also gets hot and sweaty at the least exertion. Periods are usually too heavy and too frequent, often with associated pains in the breast, which may be hard and swollen just before the period begins. A profuse milky coloured leucorrhea, worse before the flow, is also common.

Impotency with increased sexual desire is a constitutional feature. The chest is often affected with a loose cough, usually worse at night, and the chest wall painful to touch. The slightest effort of going upstairs causes shortness of breath, the legs weak and exhausted, particularly in the mornings. Dizziness and vertigo is present, worse for looking upwards as on going upstairs or for quick movements. Rheumatism and gout are seen, often right-sided, and always the cramping or drawing pains are worse for cold. Generally the skin is rough and scaly, the hands hot and damp and there is a weak passive handshake. *Calcarea* patients are thirsty, but can often feel nausea after drinking.

Modalities:

Better for: Being constipated, rest, warmth, being stroked or rubbed.

Worse for: Open air, water, bathing or washing, damp cold air, in the morning, and 2 -3 a.m., in the Autumn, any exertion.

The Kali Carb Constitution

Mentals

Tired, restless, tearful, listless, unable to sleep, particularly wakes after 4.00 a.m. Bored, irritable, lonely, intolerant of others, dislikes being left alone. Mood swings, lacking confidence, over-hasty and precipitate in actions and desicion-making. Lacks tact with others.

General Indications for Kali Carb as a remedy:

Fleshy, well-build, overweight people. Anaemic with a tendency to fluid-retention. Great exhaustion and general weakness.

Site of Action:

The mind and emotions, mucous membranes of throat, respiratory tree, digestive system, genito-urinary tract. This leads to characteristic extreme dryness and the frequent sharp cutting or stinging pains from the irritation. It also acts on the haemopoietic system, haemoglobin production and thyroid.

Symptoms:

Headache, often in the evenings, behind the eyes or of the forehead. The head is heavy, especially the left side. Upper eyelids swollen and puffy due to fluid retention in the area. Faintness. Yellow catarrh discharges, both nostrils blocked. Hay fever common. Frequent colds and sneezing, especially when out of doors. Gums bleed easily. The mouth and tongue are sore, the latter dry, having a 'dirty' taste. The throat is sore, burning, irritated, often worse in the evening and better for hot drinks. Appetite is variable, with increased thirst for hot drinks. The abdomen is bloated and there is frequent regurgitations, acid or a 'hot bubble sensation', sometimes with acute spasm. Alternating constipation and diarrhoea. Dribbling on urine, lack of libidinal drive. Asthma on retiring or during the night, waking the patient at 4.00 a.m. Intermittent daytime coughing. The limbs are tired or swollen. Pain of the large joints, especially on the left side, as the left knee or left hip. Low back pain.

Modalities:

Better for: Warm drinks, movement, warm weather, rest.

Worse for: Dust and dryness, cold, draughts and damp. For carrying or exercise. On waking, or in the late evening and early hours, 3-4.00 a.m.

The Lycopodium Constitution

Mentals:

Sensitive, shy, nervous, precocious intellectual people, often irritable, anxious, sad and depressed, weeping easily, forgetful, miserly, hypochondriacal. *Lycopodium* patients prefer solitude but are fearful of being left alone in the house. They lack confidence and are full of doubts, particularly about the future. Intellectual self-mistrust is a feature. Much of the anxiety is anticipatory in type. Often bright over-sensitive people, with a lot of ability, they are easily depressed, and particularly irritable or 'ugly' on waking. May become anorexic and preoccupied with body image as part of their hypochondriasis. At times they get confused, use wrong words and make mistakes in handwriting.

General Indications:

Dark complexioned, sensitive intellectuals, weak in muscular development, dry skinned, thin, looking prematurely old. Particularly problems of the gastro-intestinal tract when there is flatulence, right-sided burning pains, constipation, and the typical *Lycopodium* anxiety.

Site of Action:

Lycopodium affects the body generally in a deep way – for a period of about eight weeks. It particularly affects the gastro-intestinal tract, especially the large intestine. Liver, soft tissues, blood vessels, bones and joints.

Symptoms:

Facial neuralgia, right-sided and burning. Thirst for drinks, little and often. Styes. Dryness of mucous membrane and skin. *Lycopodium* patients rarely sweat. Vaginal dryness, also of the eyes which are sticky in the morning, red and ulcerated. Photophobia. Nasal catarrh, worse in the right nostril. The gastric symptoms are marked with great hunger, but immediately full after a few mouthfuls, and a weak sinking giddy sensation if a meal is delayed or missed. Sourness burning pains, indigestion, the abdomen very sensitive to pressure or touch. There is tenderness in the right upper abdomen and liver and they cannot lie on the right side at night. The right chest is also tender, also right-sided tonsillitis, right-sided sciatica.

Hernia. Constipation. Vertigo on getting up. Burning pains in the right arm. *Lycopodium* patients are unable to wear tight clothing, as it worsens the abdominal discomfort. Renal colic often right-sided with red sand in the urine and renal stones, urine slow to flow. Haemorrhoids. There is a dry tickling cough, shortness of breath and a salty grey phlegm is coughed up. Viral pneumonia – particularly of the right lung base. Warts on the hands. The onset of periods is frequently too early and profuse. They usually crave sweet foods. The right foot feels hot and the left one is cold. Lumbago, chronic gouty rheumatism, eczema of the scalp, the skin may ulcerate.

Modalities:

Better for: Cool open air, warmth, motion, uncovering, warm drinks.

Worse for: Oysters, being in public, afternoon 4-8 p.m. pressure.

The Natrum Mur Constitution

Mentals:

Natrum mur people are very nice to know, but are changeable and difficult to treat. Their mood varies from one moment to the next, from nervous excitement and laughter to tears, depression, anxiety or despair. They often feel resentful and disappointed, without much sense of humour, so that they quickly become irritable and frustrated. Over sensitive, they are of a solitary make-up, worse for consolation, soothing or handling, hating fuss or attention of any kind. They are often awkward and hasty, hypochondrical, ill at ease and tense, rarely able to be natural in any social situation. Grief and mourning.

General Indications:

The nervousness of the mental make-up, craving for salt, dryness of the mucous membranes, weakness, chilly but intolerant of heat.

Site of Action:

Natrum mur acts profoundly on the body generally, with especial action on the skin, intestine, and mucous membranes of the body.

Symptoms:

Tired, chilly, exhausted, weak, knees, legs and feet are very cold, oedematous face, on a thin body. Cold sores of the lips and nose, the lips body. Cold sores of the lips and nose, the lips cracked in the corners, the lower lip with a deep furrowed long-standing soreness and cracking. The whole lower lip may become swollen, urticarial and develop a large blister followed by scab formation. These is a loss of taste and smell, with chronic nasal catarrh, dryness in the throat and also of the vagina, with painful intercourse, frigidity and spasm. The anal area is also dry with anal fissuring.

Constipation is a feature with the painful passage of hard, dry, crumbling stools, with bleeding, soreness and tearing pains when first passed, and a feeling of retention of the stool. Anaemia, shortness of breath and weakness on climbing stairs, with palpitation, cardiac weakness or degenerations, tightness in the chest and missed heart beats with an irregular pulse. Indigestion with nausea, heartburn, a distended stomach, hunger. There is loss of weight.

The tongue is red, shining, with irregular areas of shape or mapping, clean, with a numb heaviness. Blisters may be present on the tongue, or herpes infection and eruptions around the mouth, hair-line and anal region. There is a bitter taste in the mouth, the skin is greasy and infected, particularly along the hair-line with a moist eczematous eruption. Hang nails are common. There is a white mucous leucorrhoea.

Uterine prolapse. Sterility. The periods are too early and tend to be heavy with a headache, both before and after the flow. The headaches are throbbing and bursting, usually over the forehead, worse on waking, (*Natrum* patients having a tendency to early morning waking), and lasting through the day, aggravated by coughing or concentration. The eyes weep profusely from exposure to cold wind when walking. Cramps of the throat, rectum and uterus are common. There is always a craving for salt, and an aggravation of all symptoms from the seaside, although in some there is an improvement.

The urinary tract is involved with delayed starting of the flow, especially when others are present. Involuntary leaking, and burning pains in the urethra after micturition. Often there is chronic oedema of the legs and face. Low backache is a common factor, better for pushing a firm pillow into the small of the back or for lying on a firm bed. Epilepsy. Chills, intermittent fever, and sweats may occur.

Modalities:

Better for: Open air, continued movement and walking, fasting, empty stomach, backache better for firm local pressure and a hard bed.

Worse for: Consolation, heat, the sun, sea air, the damp, mornings 10-11 a.m., headaches worse for coughing, music, heat.

The Nux Vomica Constitution

Mentals:

Irritable, angry, impulsive to violence or suicide, excessively sensitive and intense people, easily offended. Depressed but quickly resentful, hasty and cross, malicious, spiteful and passionately involved with causes. Tense, determined and tenacious, fastidious, particularly highly-pressurized office and business workers in sedentary occupations. Addicted to work, coffee, taking excess alcohol and stimulants generally – living 'on their nerves'. There is obsessional fear of knives.

General Indications:

Usually thin people with dark hair and complexion. Whenever there is the combination of spasm, tension and hypersensitivity with constipation, pain, association with headache, indigestion and the *Nux vomica* mentality.

Site of Action:

The mind and central nervous system, gastro-intestinal tract, circulation, and all the voluntary muscles of the body.

Symptoms:

The *Nux vomica* patient is chilly, craving heat, the whole body cold even when feverish, the face usually burning red. There is a tendency for spasm and tension, both in the mind and body generally, with pain and colic of bladder, rectum, kidney, gall bladder, intestine, oesophagus and uterus. Constipation is a feature, due to irregular peristalsis, with a constant desire to pass a motion, but weak and ineffective, so that the stool cannot be evacuated. It may be blood-stained from piles, and there is a tendency to faint or vomit after the attempted bowel movement.

Prolapse of the uterus or rectum, or inguinal, umbilical or hiatus hernia. The *Nux vomica* patient faints easily – from odours, in a warm room, from belching, after eating, in labour, from emotion. Indigestion is a marked feature, with a heavy weight-like feeling, one to two hours after eating, with a sour taste, swollen and bloated upper abdomen, and intolerance to tight clothes. Hiccough and nausea, particularly nausea of pregnancy are common. The periods are painful, with irregular cramping pains, too early and too heavy, the flow dark. There may be flooding. Labour pains are intense and may provoke fainting. The nipples are sore when nursing. Premature ejaculation may be a problem. Headache is a feature – worse from anger, coughing and thunder. The *Nux vomica* backache is constant, bruised, burning and tearing, usually in the low back, with inability to turn over in bed – the patient has to sit up in order to change position.

Modalities:

Better for: Gentle rain, sleep, eating fats, heat, hot drinks, warm wet weather.

Worse for: Dry or windy weather, winter, jarring, touch, noise, odours, uncovering, draughts, morning, eating, concentration, anger, after midnight and before 2-3.00 a.m., open air. The heat of the bed aggravates.

The Phosphorus Constitution

Mentals:

Hypersensitive, anxious, needing reassurance and company. Very sensitive to atmospherics, such as storms, thunder and the dark. Fears being alone, thunder, death. Bright, eager, intelligent, enthusiastic, they feel better for being touched or massaged. Often excitable, with vivid thoughts and imaginations, at other times withdrawn, indifferent, silent or apathetic. Can be very difficult, angry and irritable with the family. Sadness with a need for attention, to be reassured is a strong feature, don't take their eyes off you. Easily startled. Exhausted.

General Indications:

Often tall, thin stooping spine, red-haired people, with sallow, waxy skin and delicate eyelashes. Burning left-sided pains, diarrhoea, weakness, perspiration, chest problems, usually right-sided, restless, bleeding is a frequent feature.

Site of Action:

The body generally, has a strong action on the bones, circulations, liver, heart, pancreas, gastro-intestinal tract, and respiratory tract. Central nervous system.

Symptoms:

Nervous, weak, often tired with violent hunger and a thirst for cold drinks. Burning pains in the stomach and chest are common. Wounds bleed and bruise easily. The chest is affected with a dry hacking cough, shortness of breath, hoarseness, asthma, pleurisy, right-sided pneumonia, the abdomen distended. Typhoid fever, yellow fever, typhus, fainting, sweats, intermittent fever, burning pains everywhere, with sinking fainting feelings. Anaemia, jaundice.

There is a watery offensive diarrhoea with pale greenish stool. Vomiting. Nausea of pregnancy, vomiting after anaesthetics. The periods are too early and scanty, or absent with vicarious bleeding, such as nose-bleeds. Leucorrhoea. Pain in the left ovary. The breasts have burning pains. *Phosphorus* cannot get off to sleep, insomnia is a problem, and they sleep usually on the right side. There is a bead of sweat on the upper lip. Salt is craved, as also *cold* drinks and ice cream. Often hungry at night but tired, weak, yet with constant urgent hunger and thirst. There is a twitching of muscles, paralysis, epilepsy, hemiplegia.

Modalities:

Better for: Sleep, eating, warmth, massage, lying on the right side, cold drinks and applications, fresh air.

Worse for: Touch, lying on the left side, thunderstorm, damp or hot weather, exertion.

The Pulsatilla Constitution

Mentals:

Mild and yielding personality, easily moved emotionally to tears or laughter. Gentle, changeable disposition, sad, depressed, hypochondrical, usually good-tempered, but can also be tiresome and demanding. Irritable, restless, demanding sympathy and attention. Slow, placid.

General Indication:

Fair or sandy-haired, blue-eyed, pale, rather plump people. Indigestion, respiratory infections, often with catarrh or period problems. The symptoms are usually worse at night and aggravated by heat.

Site of Action:

The body generally, but particularly circulatory system and kidneys with retention of fluid and overloading of the circulations, respiratory and gastro-intestinal tracts, genital organs. Affects the large joints of the body.

Symptoms:

There is congestion of nose and throat with a profuse varied thick-yellow-green catarrh. The mouth is dry, the tongue covered with a sticky mucous, eyes red and inflamed, with styes, the lower lid particularly inflamed, itchy and sticky. Vision is dimmed and there is a profuse

217

watery discharge. The throat is sore and congested, ears painful with violent pains and a yellow discharge, deafness, scarlet fever. Toothache is worse for warm drinks, food and in the evening, better for cool air and uncovering. There is often a cough, dry, raw, painful, the air passages blocked by an excess of mucous, with thick yellow or green phlegm produced. All symtoms worse at night and for heat and warmth. *Pulsatilla* patients sweat profusely. Vertigo when sitting and tinnitus – the noises like a roaring sound. All symptoms are changeable and vary from day to day. Indigestion is common, food tastes bitter, and there is rumbling colic, griping pains and abdominal heaviness, worse one hour after food, with flatulence and heartburn. Diarrhoea with watery green mucous stool. Haemorrhoids and varicose veins. Frequent passing of water, particularly at night. The testicles may be swollen with hydrocele. Periods are absent, delayed or scanty. There is painless leucorrhoea – with a thick milky mucous discharge. The skin is burning, itching and uncomfortable, worse in the evening. Rheumatism a feature, particularly of the knee joints. Anxiety is worse in the evening, with restlessness, inability to fall asleep, feeling too hot under the covers, needing to put the feet out of the bed. Often they feel thirsty at about 2.00 a.m., and get up to pass water and either walk around or make a cup of tea and eat a biscuit.

Modalities:

Better for: Cool, open fresh air, cold food and cold applications, uncovering, slow easy movement, consolation and sympathy.

Worse for: A warm room, heat, hot bath, closed stuffy room, in the evening, fats and rich foods.

The Sepia Constitution

Mentals:

Irritable, sad, depressed and exhausted. All
affection is diminished, indifferent to others,
even their own family and those loved best.
There is an absence of joy, intolerant, dull, lazy,
sometimes deluded. They dislike parties and
social situations and company generally, but
enjoy dancing. Resentful, miserly, spiteful and
obstinate, with a 'martyr' like attitude at
times. They tend to be envious of others and in-
dependent, not wanting to be helped and re-
jecting. The two main anxiety areas are
poverty and things getting worse. They may be
weepy in the evenings, but often *Sepia* constitutions want to cry but are unable to, and
when they do cry they feel better for it. They
may be restless and excitable but usually are
languid, apathetic and lazy, tending to look for
solitude and are taciturn. Often fearful of
ghosts.

General Indications:

The *Sepia* person is rather puffy and flabby,
dark haired, with a yellow sallow skin and
brownish-yellow blotches and spots on the skin
and in the saddle area across the nose, tall with
a long back. The skin is cold, damp and may be
freckled. Exhaustion, irritability, indigestion,
and genito-urinary problems.

Site of Action:

Particularly the genital organs, bladder, gastro-intestinal tract, skin and respiratory tract.

Symptoms:

The scalp itches, the hair thin and falling out. Brownish warts on the neck. The uterus is strangely affected with prolapse, pressing down pains, or the sensation of a lump in the vagina, so that the patient sits with legs crossed to prevent the whole uterus 'falling' out of the body. Periods tend to be scanty and too early, but sometimes late, and profuse at times. There is an unpleasant acrid yellowish leucorrhoea, the vagina dry. Dragging down dysmennor- hoea, itching in the vaginal vulval area, hot flushes of the menopause. Nausea of preg- nancy, morning sickness. Abortion.

Constipation is a feature usually in the morning with weak upset stomach and bearing down abdominal pains into the pelvis. The bladder is irritated, with frequent passage of a thick offensive slimy yellowish urine. Noc- turnal enuresis, especially just after first falling asleep. The liver is enlarged, congested and tender. Haemorroids. The *Sepia* patient feels as if there is a ball or hard lump in the rectum or vagina, pressing and pushing down. There may be a history of fibroids. There is usually aversion to the opposite sex and com- plete disinterest in sexuality. Impotence.

Hunger is gnawing and acute for spicy foods, but with intolerance of fats. Hunger is not relieved by eating. Catarrh is a feature of chest, throat, eyes, nose, vagina, and genito-urinary system. Headache is common, usually worse in the mornings, better for eating, or quick walking. *Sepia* faints easily, particularly from standing. All discharges are offensive, such as the stool and urine. There is chronic tired low back pain, better for exercise and local pressure. Irritable over-sensitivity to smell, light and noise.

Modalities:

Better for: Rest, quick rapid movements of walking or dancing, weeping, sleep, the back for local pressure.

Worse for: Heat, change of weather, during pregnancy, during a period, thunder, eating, in the mornings, consolations.

The Silicea Constitution

Mentals:

Lacks stamina, grit and determination, weak, tired, embarrassed, yielding, no confidence, fearing failure. Dread of undertaking anything, like examinations, in case of failure. Sad, irritable, nervous, over-sensitive with rigid obsessional fixed ideas – as counting pins. Can also be very stubborn, self-willed, obstinate and touchy at times.

General Indications:

Thin, pale, listless, weak, with fine bone structure, of fair complexion. Chilly, weak, perspiring, with infection, usually with the formation of discharging pus from the skin or some other area of the body.

Site of Action:

Connective tissue, skin, lymphatic glands, respiratory and gastro-intestinal tract.

Symptoms:

Infection with suppuration and offensive discharge is characteristic. The skin has recurrent boils, ulcers, hang nail infection and is unhealthy, rough and cracked especially at the finger tips, the nails weak, rough, yellow, and breaking easily.

Perspiration is profuse, on the forehead, hands and feet with a 'wet stocking' sensation, the sweat offensive, chilly, although at times in a warm room the hands may be warm and very moist. The lips are cracked and rough.

Chill is a feature – *Silicea* patients are cold, even in a warm room, yet like cold foods as ice-cream, and feel better for them, aggravated by heat and warmth. This aggravation by heat is similar to *Pulsatilla* - and *Silicea* is always regarded as its chronic remedy. Headache is common beginning at the back of the head and moving forward over the skull to settle in the forehead, or over the right eye, with persistent severe tearing pains, better for local pressure, wrapping up the head, and for urination. *Silicea* acts strongly on foreign bodies, as a splinter in the finger. It also reduces the hardness and induration of scar tissue generally. Circulation is erratic and varied with hot flushes of blood to the head, but chilly cold extremities with the fingers and toes white, bloodless, wrinkled and 'dead'. The abdomen is hard, tense, swollen, with offensive flatus. Constipation is usual with a hard small lumpy stool – only partly expelled and partly retained in the rectum – the 'bashful' stool.

The breast is often hard, red and tender from abcess formation after mastitis, the nipple inverted and funnel-like. There may be vaginal discharge of blood occuring on breast feeding. Impotence. Vertigo – worse from looking upward. The lymph nodes are often enlarged, tender and may suppurate or discharge. Gums are tender, soft, infected, the teeth yellow and decayed. The tongue has a sensation – as if there were a hair on it. Paralysis. Epilepsy. Fissure-in-ano, rectal fissures.

Modalities:

Better for: Cool air, cold food and cold applications, massage, binding the head tightly.

Worse for: Cold, uncovering at night, a new or full moon, lying on the left side, milk.

The Sulphur Constitution

Mentals:

A disordered, confused, untidy mind and body. The 'ragged' philosopher, scholar, inventor. Anxious about small minor matters, depressed or unconcerned, and everything pleases, even rags are beautiful. Irritable and impatient at times, nervous and restless.

General Indications:

Sulphur looks untidy – winding a scarf around the neck whether it is needed or not – red-faced and is clumsy, lean, stooping, restless, covered with a dirty-looking infective skin which has boils and eruptions with discharging pustules, vesicles and eczematous areas.

Relapsing complaints which do not respond to apparently well indicated remedies, in particular there are burning infective areas of the skin, and burning pains in all areas of the body.

Site of Action:

The skin, circulation, gastro-intestinal tract, genito-urinary tract, the reactive powers of the body generally.

Symptoms:

Redness and itching is characteristic of the face, eyelids, particularly the nose, but also lips, and anal-vulval area, the orifices are red, congested, swollen and sore. The top of the head is hot and there is a sick headache – worse after eating. Hot flushes are common, particularly at the menopause. Menorrhagia. The periods are late and irregular. There is ravenous appetite. The *Sulphur* person eats everything as if starved, and likes sweet foods, savouries, and salt, particularly rich fatty creams and butter. Milk usually disagrees and causes vomiting. There is chronic indigestion and constipation with diarrhoea – worse in the early morning about 5.00-6.00 a.m. that drives them out of bed to pass a loose very offensive stool.

Alcoholism. Tuberculosis. Ankle oedema. The top of the head is hot, the feet cold. Pneumonia, asthma, cough. Frequent urination, impotence. There is a characteristic empty 'sinking' feeling in the stomach about 11.00 a.m., with great hunger and a compulsion to eat. The tongue is coated, stomach distended, with griping pains, after little food, and there is burning in the rectum and anus – with the passage of a foul rotten egg-smelling flatus. The feet are usually pushed out of the bed at night.

Modalities:

Better for: Movement, scratching.

Worse for: Rest, standing, heat, the sun, milk, washing, bathing and water generally, heat of the bed, after sleep, after eating.

The Thuja Constitution

Mentals:

Depressed, and irritable, scrupulous, acts and talks quickly, in a hurry. Aphasia. Mistakes are made with words, especially in writing – when letters are missed or in speech when words are left out. Anxious, weeps easily, worse for music. Mental subnormality. Can be very difficult people to live with because of ill-humour, peevish demands and irritability. There are many delusional features. The upper part of the body feels brittle and made of glass. A sensation of a live animal in the abdomen. Headaches are of a nail being driven into the brain. Paranoia. Dreams of falling, or of flinging themselves from a height.

General Indications:

The *Thuja* constitution is usually under average height, has a tendency to subnormality, dark complexion, black hair, unhealthy greasy and waxy skin. Easily exhausted. The ill-effects of vaccination, polyps, warts, chronic catarrh.

Site of Action:

The body generally, particularly the skin, fibrous tissue.

Symptoms:

The characteristic symptom is a tendency to new growth, with multiple warts, polyps, fibrous tumours, many of the warty growths have a cauliflower-like formation, soft and spongy which ooze an offensive, sweetish-smelling discharge. There is chronic catarrh of nose, chest or stomach, with asthma or gastric ulcer. The skin may also develop chilblains or a moist eczema. Headaches are frequent, often left-sided, situated in the forehead area, associated with frequency of micturition. Pains are dull like a tight hand, or as if a nail was driven through. Neuralgia of the left temple. The teeth are unhealthy, infected, with enamel defects, caries, the gums swollen, unhealthy, pyorrhoea.

The body is cold and shivery, with oily offensive sweat on the uncovered parts of the body, also in the anal-genital area with anal fissure and genital or anal warts. Periods are usually too early. Often the left ovary is painful. Abortion. Urethritis, prostatis, leucorrhoea – greenish, burning excoriating discharge. Varicocoele. The urine stream is forked or delayed. Bladder paralysis. The *Thuja* patient usually has a capricious appetite, takes no breakfast, but drinks too much tea. The left testicle is painful. Left-sided inquinal hernia. Diarrhoea is common – the stool watery-yellow, spluttering with much flatus. There is arthritis of the large joints.

Chapter thirty-three

Minor Constitutional Types

The Aethusa Constitution

Mentals:

The main feature is weakness of mind, and inability to think or concentrate. Confused, often mentally retarded and sleepy. At the same time there are outbursts of rage with an irritable restless anxiety and crying. These outbursts are often violent, and this is a key feature coming on with acute violent convulsion, and many of the mental and other symptoms have this feature of violent onset. With epilepsy the eyes are turned downwards and delirium and hallucinations may occur – typically seeing rats or mice running across the room.

General Indications for Aethusa as a remedy:

The main indications are the combinations of exhaustion and weakness of thought processes and the body generally combined with sudden violent symptoms particularly vomiting. There is always an absence of thirst.

Site of Action:

The remedy affects the mind and central nervous system and also the gastro-intestinal tract.

Symptoms:

Aethusa is intolerant of milk and it is useful in the vomiting of infants. The vomit is sudden, violent and a forceful projectile – as if shot from a cannon. Large amounts of yellow, sometimes green coloured curds are vomited immediately after feeding. The child falls asleep immediately after the vomiting and wakes up hungry. It is also useful in persistent vomiting in adults. Colic, diarrhoea is common with severe lancing pains and often the face is drawn with anxiety, sunken and pale looking, particularly white in the upper lip areas.

Modalities:

Better for: Being in the open fresh air, eating, morning and evening.

Worse: 3-4.00 a.m.

The Agaricus Constitution

Mentals:

Excitement, uncontrollable rage, delirium, alcoholism, dizziness, intoxication, making foolish and incoherent conversation often with ideas of power and grandeur. The elation and accompanying mirth is followed by depression and confusion.

General Indications for Agaricus as a remedy:

Confusional states, chilblains and spinal rheumatism. Epilepsy and chorea may often be relieved.

Site of Action:

Agaricus affects the central nervous system, involuntary muscles and circulation generally.

Symptoms:

There is nervous twitching of the whole body, particularly involving face, eyes, eyelids, mouth and neck. Tics are an indication. There may be head rolling. *Agaricus* has severe headache as if a nail were driven into the head – often right-sided. Symptoms occur on diagonally opposite sides of the body, as a twitching left eye and painful right knee. Circulation is severely affected with redness, burning and itching particularly on the nose, ear and feet, but with little swelling. With chilblains the extremities are blue and icy cold. Breath and stools are offensive and a lot of flatus is passed. Stitch pains in the spleen area may occur. Pain along the spinal column is severe, worse when bending down and radiates along the spine into the legs. Rheumatism in the back, feeling bruised and sprained or tearing pains in the legs. Unable to lean back in a chair as so tender. There may also be tremor of hands – worse on writing, and legs as if the limbs do not belong to them.

Modalities:

Better for: Warmth, slowly moving about.

Worse for: Cold weather, cold water, the open air, before a thunderstorm, with rest.

The Alumina Constitution

Mentals:

There is sadness, confusion, impatience and anxiety. Time passes too slowly, so that they become uneasy, impulsive and hasty. Moods are changeable and there is a tendency to hypochondriasis.

General Indications for Alumina as a remedy:

Chronic illnesses in people of sedentary occupation, there is pallor, weakness and fatigue, with marked severe constipation.

Site of Action:

Alumina affects mucous membrane of the whole body and is indicated whenever there is severe dryness of mucosa or paralysis of surrounding involuntary muscles.

Symptoms:

Constipation with considerable straining, the rectum feels paralysed, great effort and straining are needed even to pass a soft stool. Weakness, pallor, fatigue, exhaustion, fainting and anaemia is marked and there is sluggishness of the body generally – the legs in particular feel heavy and tired even when sitting – the heels numb. The throat feels dry particularly in the evening and there is either a chronic sore throat or the need to clear it frequently, with a raw dry feeling and hoarseness. The sensation is often of a splinter or fishbone caught in the throat.

The chest is also affected with a hacking chronic cough, often causing vomiting. Nasal catarrh with dryness is also common. Periods are scanty, weak, pale and often late or there may be a severe, profuse, burning leucorrhea. Pains occur in any part of the body but particularly in the low back – like a hot iron. The pains move upwards and are burning in character. The skin is unhealthy, often infected, the face feels as if covered with a cobweb. Itching and irritation occurs, worse with the heat of the bed. Squint may occur due to paralysis of one internal rectus muscle, or the lids may drop heavily. *Alumina* has strange food cravings, particularly for dry foods and there may be odd strange cravings for starch, chalk or charcoal. There is trembling weakness of the whole body with convulsions, unsteadiness and a staggering gait.

Modalities:

Better for: Avoiding aluminium kitchen utensils, warmth generally, warm food and drink and moisture.

Worse for: Cold dry air, winter, potatoes, a new or full moon.

The Antimonium Tartrate Constitution

Mentals:

They are excessively irritable, bad humoured, depressed and restless. The child cries easily, wants to be carried and does not want to be touched or examined. In addition they are drowsy, tired, prostrated, near-comatosed when more severely ill, and fearful of being alone.

General Indications for Antimonium tart. as a remedy:

Nausea, diarrhoea, collapse, coldness and pallor. The whole body covered with a chilly perspiration.

Site of Action:

The remedy acts strongly on both respiratory organs and gastro-intestinal system, affecting mucous membrane with a thick profuse catarrhal inflammation and irritation.

Symptoms:

Prostration, weakness, chill, the face pale and may be cyanosed or blue, the body covered with cold sweat. Persistent severe nausea and vomiting, often severe watery diarrhoea is characteristic. The remedy is effective in chorea. The tongue has a thick, white coating, sometimes red or dry in the middle, the tips of the papillae shining through. The chest feels constricted full and suffocating, and there is a coarse noisy rattling of mucous on breathing which cannot easily be coughed up. Anger and irritability are frequent and often provoke a bout of dry, short, ineffective coughing, which does not clear the accumulation of mucous. It is useful in pneumonia, asthma, whooping cough, and particularly in the weak child or elderly. Headache and lumbago are also common. They are typically thirstless and have aversion to all food.

Modalities:

Better for: For vomiting, and sitting upright.

Worse for: Cold, damp, also for heat, sitting forward, 4.00 a.m.

The Apis Constitution

Mentals:

Sad, tearful, depressed, *Apis* make-up is restless and fearful, needing company and does not want to be left alone. At times they are irritable and suspicious. Frequently clumsy and awkward, dropping things.

General Indications for Apis as a remedy:

Whenever there is burning, stinging pain, with redness, swelling and an absence of thirst. Restlessness is characteristic.

Site of Action:

This is very general, the brain, mind, throat, chest, intestine, anus, and genitals may all be affected.

Symptoms:

The characteristic picture is of stinging irritations, pain, with a bruised feeling and great sensitivity to touch. Every hair is painful. Exhaustion is common, and the *Apis* patient is always sleepy, frequently yawning when awake. Sleep restless, or may be deeply comatosed. There is restless fidgeting, twitching and jerking. Stiffness accompanies the swelling – of jaws, throat, tongue, chest, and may paralyse speech or constrict breathing, so that there is a dry hacking cough, the face red or purple. Burning heat without thirst is a feature – and may affect the eyes, ears, throat, chest, abdomen, and the anus.

Swelling oedema is seen with bag-like swellings under the eyes. The ankles may be swollen, the thoracic or abdominal cavities full of fluid which is painless. Everywhere there is a tight, tense feeling, particularly the feet feel too large, swollen and stiff. Diarrhoea, with involuntary loss of stool, the anus feels open raw and stinging. Hemiplegia, paralysis, meningitis associated with a loud piercing cry – often when sleeping. The skin is usually white and transparent, under tension, because of the oedema. Urticaria and erisipelas both respond well to *Apis*.

Modalities:

Better for: Cold water, pressure locally on the head area.

Worse for: Heat, touch, tight clothing, pressure.

The Argentum Nitricum Constitution

Mentals:

The *Argentum* person is highly nervous, shaking, quick and impulsive, always in a hurry, full of irrational fears, panics, obsessions and preoccupations. They fear death and experience considerable anticipatory anxiety before examinations, or any public performance. Time passes slowly so that they cannot wait to get everything over and done with, always frustrated and anxious, rushing at whatever they do, so that their efforts often lead to failure. Agoraphobia. Epilepsy is common, especially when following a fright or associated with the menstrual cycle – the pupils characteristically dilated before the onset of an attack.

General Indications for Argentum nitricum as a remedy:

Restless anxiety and panic, in a warm person who rarely feels cold and suffers most intensely from the heat.

Site of Action:

Apart from the acute main symptoms, the mucous membranes of the body may be affected generally with inflammation, ulceration and irritation – particularly involving eyes, throat, stomach and intestines.

Symptoms:

There is considerable general exhaustion,
weakness and tremor. Throat symptoms are
common with thick mucous and splinter-like
pain. The eyes are commonly affected with
conjunctivitis – acute and catarrhal, or
ulcerative symptoms with a purulent discharge. Serpent-like 'floaters' are a feature
when looking upwards. The tip of the tongue is
red and painful. Headache is common – generalised or in the left, frontal region. The head
feels swollen and enlarged, often relieved by
local pressure or binding the head firmly.
Diarrhoea is also a feature, spluttering, green
and watery, with colic and there is always a
great deal of noisy flatulence. The skin is dry,
withered, sometimes prematurely old, itching
and hard with a brown, blue-greenish discolouration. Sugar is craved, taken in large
amounts often leading to vomiting. In addition
they like a lot of salt.

Modalities:

Better for: Cold air or cold drinks.

Worse for: Heat in any form, either local or
general.

The Arnica Constitution

Mentals:

Nervous, frightened, over-sensitive, restless, anxious make-up, with a tendency to agoraphobia. Fearful of going out, meeting people and also hypochondriacal. Often solitary, they are reluctant to converse and are easily irritated. *Arnica* is forgetful, feels depressed and hopeless, has a poor memory and a horror of sudden death.

General Indications for Arnica as a remedy:

The best, most useful trauma and first aid remedy, dealing with symptoms of sudden onset, often where there is a history of recent emotional stress and strain. Especially indicated in well-built, ruddy-complexioned people, liable to travel-sickness who always complain that the bed is too hard, and therefore sleep fitfully. It is usually only of value during the initial six days of an acute traumatic condition, and then needs to be followed by a further remedy, if not cured.

Site of Action:

A soft tissue remedy affecting intercostal muscles of the chest wall, and surrounding fibrous tissues. It is always an acute short-acting remedy, but also helpful when a traumatic accident has occurred many years previously.

Symptoms:

Bruising, such as a black eye, pain or swelling, after trauma or muscular fatigue, rupture and spasm. Pains are stitch-like and often affect the chest, limbs and back with a pleuritic type of pain, worse for movement and pressure. It is indicated in fatigue, exhaustion, shock, loss of blood, as in cerebral haemorrhage, and also before and after tooth extraction, or any surgical or manipulative intervention, as a fracture or dislocations. The body feels weak and sluggish, the limbs heavy. There is a bruised, beaten feeling as if the affected part has been sprained or dislocated, and pains begin in the lower body and move upwards. The *Arnica* constitution often has a cold nose and body although the head feels hot. It is useful in rheumatic conditions involving the large and small joints of the body. The heart may be involved in the rheumatism as a complication.

Modalities:

Better for: Local pressure, lying on the unaffected side, lying down, rest, lying with the head low.

Worse for: Movement, walking, touch, pressure, the evening, damp, cold, lying on the affected side.

The Aurum Metallicum Constitution

Mentals:

There is profound hopelessness and depression with suicidal tendencies, a longing for death and disgust with life. At the same time they are extremely irritable, and the least contradiction or frustration causes them to fly into a rage. Sometimes extremely emotional and hysterical.

General Indications for Aurum as a remedy:

Severe depression following acute fright or shock or less often a disappointment in a romantic attachment. Depression is frequently associated with various heart or genital symptoms.

Site of Action:

Gold affects the whole organism, but in particular its actions are most marked on the mind, genital area, heart, liver, eyes and bones.

Symptoms:

It is an excellent cardiac remedy, particularly for the elderly when there is spinning dizziness or vertigo on bending down. Palpitations, congestion and chest pains referred along the arm to the fingertips. The testicles are often undeveloped in thin, pale, undersized boys, sometimes hard or undescended, the right testicle is frequently painful. The uterus is enlarged, often prolapsed, a creamy coloured leucorrhea is common. Pains in the bone occur – as in the right jaw area, the nasal bones sore and if severe and chronic, there may be infection with ulceration. The liver is often enlarged. Eye signs are characteristic and there is diminished upper visual field. They are always very chilly and feel the cold intensely.

Modalities:

Better for: Movement, walking and warmth.

Worse for: Rest, at night, and when cold.

The Baryta Carb Constitution

Mentals:

Generally there is anxiety, fear, lack of confidence and trust, particularly in strange, new situations. They are depressed, weep easily and prefer to be alone. In the elderly there are all the symptoms of senility and second childhood with impaired memory, especially for recent events, and the mind is weak in all areas and confusion common.

General Indications for Baryta Carb as a remedy:

Baryta is usually a short person, who has never attained full height and often weight for their age. It is indicated in the young child, who is small, undersized and where normal growth-milestones have not been reached. In the elderly it is an excellent remedy, the patient often fat, unsteady, sluggish and there is deterioration of both body and mind – due to hardening of the arteries.

Site of Action:

The mind and central nervous system is strongly affected, also the lymphatic system, particularly of the neck region and the throat and tonsil region. Respiratory and digestive systems, also the heart, circulation and skin.

Symptoms:

They are always chilly, sweat profusely, particularly the feet with offensive perspiration, and are particularly likely to develop infection of the tonsils and throat whenever they catch a cold. Often the right tonsil is affected, the gland swollen, enlarged and inflamed. Abcess may develop or quinsy with suppuration. It may become chronic, surrounding lymph glands swollen, tender and painful. Swallowing is painful, particularly when the mouth is empty, although it is relieved by taking soft foods.

Whenever there is an acute throat with either single or multiple swollen glands – *Baryta Carb* is indicated. It is also useful for single lumps or swellings anywhere in the body, especially if soft, large and fatty. Glandular fever is an indication. Headache, dizziness on bending, nausea, a sense of pressure on the top of the head, loss of hair and alopoecia in young people often responds well to *Baryta* – the scalp usually tender.

The nasal passages are always dry and haemorrhage before the menstrual period may occur. They sometimes have an odd symptom of smelling the odour of pine-smoke.

The tongue may be paralysed, with much salivation and dribbling. Swallowing is painful and indigestion or colic may occur, sometimes associated with enlarged, painful abdominal glands. Chronic cough, worse in the evening and if the larynx is affected there is hoarseness, which may become chronic. The typical *Baryta* child is hungry, but refuses food, is thin, loses weight, and has a round, swollen stomach. Constipation is a feature and there is moisture and soreness in the anal region. Piles may be present, typically burning and sore. Impotence, problems of an enlarged prostate, aneurism, degenerations of mind and body generally, including the heart, with palpitations, fatigue and exhaustion after slight exertion. The skin is cold, damp, often unhealthy, itching at night in bed and interfering with sleep. There are drawing, pulsating rheumatic pains, especially the back and legs.

Modalities:

Better for: Open air, warmth, movement. The cough and discomfort on swallowing are both relieved by eating soft food.

Worse for: Cold applications, draught, damp, touch, swallowing when the mouth is empty.

The Belladonna Constitution

Mentals:

Excitement and violent delirium with impulses to bite and scratch. Anger, rage, irritability are marked and there is considerable turmoil and restlessness which may lead into an epileptic attack or convulsions. There is a hypersensitivity of all the senses with intolerance of music and bright lights. Excessive talking and constant laughter alternate with violence, with confusion of thought and mind. There is fear of black shadows.

General Indications for Belladonna as a remedy:

Acute inflammatory conditions with heat, redness and throbbing pain, high fever and restless mental excitement and delirium.

Site of Action:

Belladonna affects the body generally, with specific action on the middle and outer ear, throat, oesophagus, intestine and uterine areas. The joints may be affected in rheumatic fever. It is of special value in scarlet fever and acute throat and ear infections of children.

Symptoms:

Burning heat, redness, throbbing pains and mental excitement are the characteristic symptoms, with severe pains which suddenly come and go, worse for the least movement or jarring. They are chilly, sensitive to cold or draughts particularly when the head is uncovered or after a hair cut. Stabbing, throbbing, pulsating, burning pains, stitch-like, which are variable, come and go, in particular headache – of the forehead region, pressure-like, and worse for bending or downward movement.

The head is very sensitive and pressure on a hair may cause pain. The eyes are nearly always wide open, fixed and often staring, with dilated pupils and a bright sparkling appearance. There is often a burning heat in the eyes, the visual field has a red glow and they may see sparks before the eyes. The face is red, hot, often swollen and burning, although there is usually a pale white circular area around the mouth and chin. The tongue is dark red often with a thick white coated centre, mouth and throat are dry and swallowing is painful.

There may be a painful middle or outer ear infection with fever, violent tearing pains and restlessness. The chest may be affected with a short dry cough. Nausea and lower abdominal pains, as gall-stone colic are frequent – the whole area sore and tender to touch. The bowels are usually constipated, the stool a chalky colour. The pulse is characteristically full, rapid and forceful. The *Belladonna* patient always sweats profusely on the covered parts of the body. It is a right-sided remedy with burning, tearing, rheumatic pains in the shoulder, hands and fingers. Epilepsy may occur with spasms and convulsions and they tend to fall backwards. Periods are often heavy and early, dark in colour. It is helpful in sunstroke, *Belladonna* patients are usually thirstless.

Modalities:

Better for: Warmth, rest, quiet, bending backwards, lying on the opposite side of the painful area. Eating lemons. For covering and lying in the semi-erect position with the head fairly high.

Worse for: Touch, draught, cold, pressure, motion, jarring, noise, light, night and 4.00 p.m. Also aggravated from having their hair cut, or stooping, bending down, lying on the inflamed side.

The Benzoic Acid Constitution

Mentals:

Depression with anxiety of unpleasant things, and intolerant of deformity causing a shudder of displeasure.

General Indications for Benzoid acid as a remedy:

The remedy has a wide variety of action, but the leading indication is the passing of small amounts of dark, strong-smelling urine with a characteristic odour of horse's urine. This may be associated with painful rheumatism, chest-disease or diarrhoea.

Site of Action:

The centre of action is kidney and bladder, intestine, heart, chest, throat and joints.

Symptoms:

The patient is chilly, passes scanty urine which is deep brown or reddish coloured, offensive and very strongly smelling of horse's urine because of the high uric acid content. In dribbling of old men with prostatic problems it has proved useful. Diarrhoea – particularly in children is common, with a light, soap-like stool which is exhausting. The tongue is deeply cracked, ulcerated and spongy. There is often the sensation of a lump in the throat improved by eating. Asthma, with a dry cough, quinsy, bronchitis or pneumonia. Rheumatism and gout are a common feature, the joints crack on movement, and the pains shift, moving from left to right, often in the heart or chest area with palpitations. Pains are severe, tearing, stitch-like and paralysing, often affecting the big toe with severe gout. The wrists and fingers are swollen, weak and lack strength. Ganglion of the wrist. Bunion is a feature, prolapsed uterus. Sweating is profuse.

Modalities:

Better for: Warmth, eating.

Worse for: Open air, wine, at night, movement, uncovering, lying on the right side.

The Borax Constitution

Mentals:

Irritable, over-sensitive, frightened, anxious, wants to be held and then not. Loud noises as a cough or sneeze cause them to start or cry, tendency to be lazy, and sit around, at other times they become restless. Anxious and intolerant of downward movement, and fear of going downstairs, falling, heights, or being put back in the cot or bed having been held. The aggravation by downward movement comes into sea and air-sickness when the acute falling sensation of an air pocket or wave causes violent sickness, anxiety and discomfort. They cling very tightly when afraid.

General Indications for Borax as a remedy:

The most clear-cut indications are the very characteristic *Borax* complaint of disliking heights, the fear of falling or resentment and dislike in children of being put down. Over-sensitive to noise, causing them to jump or start is the other key indications. Usually fair-haired with a dry, loose, wrinkled skin.

Site of Action:

This is very general, but particularly involves the central nervous system, ears and inner ear balance centres, respiratory tract, and serous membrane of chest. Also breast, urinary and genital organs.

Symptoms:

Borax is pale and flabby, often with a peculiar cobweb sensation on the face. Salivation is marked with a sore, infected mouth, and white spots on the tongue and mouth, due to herpes infection. The nose is also infected and ulcerated with a dry crusty catarrh, and the external ear may discharge. There are many feeding difficulties, a child may refuse the breast when feeding. Sometimes the mouth of the infant feels burning hot.

Generally the breasts are worse after the feed when empty and more comfortable for pressure and binding. There may be acute digestive upsets, as diarrhoea, the stools yellow, green and soft. The chest is often affected with dry, hacking cough, and a sticking, pleurisy type of pain in the upper, right chest – worse for coughing and deep breathing. The phlegm expectorated has a mouldy smell or taste and is offensive.

Leucorrhea is frequent, the discharge clear and seems to feel warm. There are many urinary symptoms, particularly urethritis – the urine burning hot before and during the passage of urine. The child screams out just before micturition. Sleep is disturbed, they often wake about 3.00 a.m. from a dream, with a start or cry, and want to be lifted up or held.

Modalities:

Better for: Being held and carried, for rest, walking in the fresh air.

Worse for: Cold, wet, any downward movement, from eating fruit.

The Cantharis Constitution

Mentals:

Difficult, excited, irritable, as if intoxicated, uneasy, restless and complaining. Outbursts of anger and rage are characteristic to the point of delirium. There is heightened sexual desire.

General Indications for Cantharis as a remedy:

Burning pains of the urinary tract, skin and intestine.

Site of Action:

Acts on the body generally, but particularly affects the whole of the mucous membrane lining to the alimentary tract, from mouth to rectum. The genito-urinary and respiratory organs are also in an inflammatory condition, with increased mucosal discharge.

Symptoms:

Violent burning cutting pains of the bladder, with a burning irritation felt in the urethra. Urine is passed a few drops at a time and is agonising, or there may be urinary frequency. Urgency with a frequent desire to pass small amounts of a 'red-hot' urine which contains blood. The stomach is inflamed with burning pains, colic, and diarrhoea with violent, rectal spasm, mucous and blood in the stool. There is always thirst but no desire for drinking. The eyes may be affected, bright, pupils widely dilated, the visual field yellow. The mouth, throat, larynx, stomach and peritoneum may be involved with soreness and acute, sudden burning pains and inflammation. In bronchitis there is a thick, ropey, sticky, profuse mucous discharge, often associated with bladder symptoms. There are many skin indications, large, burning, itching and intensely painful blobs or blisters as in erisipelas, shingles, gangrene after a burn or scald.

Modalities:

Better for: Warmth, rubbing.

Worse for: Cold water, food, tobacco, coffee, drinking, bright lights.

The Carbo Veg Constitution

Mentals:

The mind like the body is sluggish, slow, indolent, inert to the point of appearing stupid. There is mental weakness and exhaustion, indifference or sometimes irritability, but always an absence of restlessness, the patient lies or sits immobile. They are also depressed, miserable and easily discouraged, fearing the dark, lacking fight or determination to resist illness.

General Indications for Carbo veg as a remedy:

Coldness, sweating, with sluggishness in everything, both mentally and physically, especially of the circulations and digestive system.

Site of Action:

The mind, circulation and mucous membrane of the body generally, particularly respiratory, digestive tract and bladder.

Symptoms:

Carbo veg is a remedy for weak, thin, exhausted conditions often for the elderly. Anaemia, worn out, lacking in vital reaction and ability to regain health and strength after a prolonged, debilitating illness. Everywhere is the slow sluggish reaction which is characteristic. There is a slow venous return to the heart with venous congestion, blue, numb, swollen, cold legs, knees and feet, covered with an icy sweat. Haemorrhoids, varicose veins, ulcers of the legs and gangrene, the exremities black. Coldness is prominent – the face pale and anaemic, covered with a sweat, the breath cold – the least effort causing collapse and weakness. Burning pains are common particularly in the chest and abdomen. Flatulence is a feature – the upper abdomen worse on lying down, the digestion weak. An offensive flatus is passed. Generally they are intolerant of fats, milk, and crave sweet or salty foods which are poorly digested. The mucous membrane of the body generally is weak, soft, tender, spongy and broken down, so that bleeding is common – with nose bleeds, haemorrhage from the stomach, bowels, bladder or gums. There is a marked absence of thirst.

Infection is common – of the throat and larynx with sore throat and hoarseness. Cough is worse from cold air, and burning pains in the chest are also complained of. Bronchitis, asthma, pneumonia, particularly of the elderly, may occur. The gums are painful, spongy and bleeding, the teeth loose. Fevers such as cholera or typhoid may occur in the tropics. There is an unpleasant leucorrhoea, burning, acid and excoriating, often associated with anal or vulval irritation. Generally the menses are early and heavy. In the evening they develop sweaty, burning feet and tend to want the windows wide open, craving oxygen and air.

Modalities:

Better for: Fresh air, fanning, sweet foods, morning, rest, sitting up in bed.

Worse for: Heat, darkness, damp cold, evening air, lying down flat, 4.00 p.m. to 11.00 p.m., fats.

The Causticum Constitution

Mentals:

Timid, anxious, weak, nervous, fearful of the future. Plagued by depression and inappropriate guilt feelings, pessimistic, mistrustful, silent, disinclined to work, lies in bed. They are restless in mind and body, tossing and turning at night, with an absence of general interest. In their relationships with others they are often extremely sensitive and very sympathetic. They tend to be clumsy.

General Indications for Causticum as a remedy:

The appearance is of a pale, thin, sallow, dejected face, and an enlarged abdomen. Weakness and paralysis of throat and neck, usually associated with urinary problems, arthritis which is deforming, and a feeling of relief from rain.

Site of Action:

The action is a very general one, particularly on mucous membrane and the muscles of throat and larynx are strongly affected, also facial jaw and neck muscles. There is nearly always involvement of the bladder and weakness.

Symptoms:

Causticum acts most strongly on the face, neck and jaw areas with weakness or paralysis of the eyelids with drooping or a tendency to close them. The tongue, one side of the face – as in Bell's palsy, or the larynx may be affected. Also the neck with torticollis or wry neck, all worse from exposure to cold draughts. At the same time there is a hyper-excitability generally, with nervous twitching, tics, chorea, epilepsy and restlessness. The tongue has a central red area with surrounding white sides.

Burning, stinging pains are present in the stomach, larynx with hoarseness or loss of voice, a dry cough. The eyes are often dry and stinging aggravated by light, the vision hazy or misty – as with cataract. The skin similarly feels dry, hot and eczamatous, particularly on the scalp. Warts on the nose are seen where the remedy is indicated. Rheumatic pains are present in the jaw which is stiff, clicks and is painful.

This rheumatic tendency is found in severe, painful, deforming arthritis of the wrists and fingers, with contracture and dull drawing pains. Urinary symptoms are a key, diagnostic feature and rarely absent. Usually there is infection with urgent desires and a difficult, frequent passage of urine, with a lack of sensation or urine flow. Involuntary leaking or dribbling is common and follows coughing or blowing the nose, laughing, crying or hurrying. Noctural enuresis can occur, usually during the first deep sleep. Paralysis of the bladder with retention of urine may also occur post-operatively.

Constipation is common – the straining only relieved by standing up to pass a stool covered with mucous. Piles are painful, sore, raw and burning, worse for walking or sitting. Dizziness and vertigo are seen, with a tendency to fall either sideways or forwards. This is often associated with progressive deafness and tinnitus, when sounds seem too loud or to re-echo unpleasantly. The periods are early and excessive, the nursing mother loses milk in sleep or when an effort is made. *Causticum* is useful after a history of the patient never well since a scald or burn often many years previously.

Modalities:

Better for: Warmth, rain and damp weather, cold drinks.

Worse for: Dryness, sweet foods, the dark, evening.

The Chamomilla Constitution

Mentals:

There is an excessive, sudden irritability, with cross, demanding, spiteful behaviour, yet desiring sympathy and associated with restlessness. Sullen anger and refusal to speak – the child whines and cries until carried and starts whenever there is any move to put him down again. Questions are resented and there is an absence of any fear of death or dying – at times, and especially when depressed, pleading for it to give relief from their suffering.

General Indications for Chamomilla as a remedy:

Teething problems of the young, acute diarrhoea, problems of pregnancy or meno-pause, with characteristic irritability, often they are fair-haired, prone to excessive coffee drinking.

Site of Action:

Mucous membrane, gums, teeth, intestinal tract, bronchial tubes and uterus.

Symptoms:

Pain when teething is a key indication, the child irritable, feverish, cross and crying, only quiet and sleeping when carried. The pains seem unbearable and worsened by anything warm as a hot drink or room. Often one cheek is red, the other pale, but generally the child is hot and sweaty. The teeth often feel too long. *Chamomilla* patients are over-sensitive to any form of pain and quite unable to tolerate it with any tranquillity of mind, good humour or fortitude. They are almost demented by it, totally exhausted and prostrated. Pain seems to dominate them, preventing sleep. Anger is such that it has a psychological effect on the whole of the intestinal system, and colic, jaundice, diarrhoea, convulsion may occur.

The typical *Chamomilla* stool feels hot and is yellow-green, watery and offensive, smelling of bad eggs. Colic, flatulence and abdominal swelling are associated. Heat is a feature with high temperature and a hot sweat on the head, face, hands and also soles of the feet which burn intensely, especially at night from the heat of the bed so that they have to be put outside the covers. They are typically hot and thirsty. Colds, coughs and catarrh are common, the breath offensive, the tongue with a thick coating, the cough usually loose, rattling, full of mucous and suffocating – worse for a warm room at night. There is frequently a characteristic numbness associated with *Chamomilla* pain. Periods are always heavy, offensive, associated with drawing labour-like pains and dark clots may be passed. In labour the pains feel unbearable and there may be threatened abortion. Anger is at times of such uncontrollable severity. Leucorrhea is a frequent problem, with a clear discharge which burns and excoriates the skin.

Modalities:

Better for: Being carried if a child, fresh air, walking touch.

Worse for: Heat, warm food, lying in bed, being covered, music, wind, damp, in the evening before midnight.

The Chelidonium Constitution

Mentals:

Fatigue, anxiety, hypochondriasis, weakness, fatigue and drowsiness.

General Indication for Chelidonium as a remedy:

Chelidonium is indicated in liver disorders and right-sided pains of the body generally, associated with liver dysfunction.

Site of Action:

The liver, spleen, kidney, lungs, intestine, joints, and circulatory system. *Chelidonium* is predominantly a right-sided remedy.

Symptoms:

The patient is tired, sleepy, jaundiced with a thin, sallow, dirty yellow skin and brightly flushed cheeks. The eyes are yellow. Dull heavy 'bruised' pains are present particularly under the right shoulder blade. There are also neuralgic pains in the right jaw, cheek, eye, and forehead. The tongue has a thick yellow coating with red edges and there is a bitter taste in the mouth. Nausea may be present with pain in the upper abdominal area referred to the back and across the umbilicus. The liver is tender and may be enlarged. The stools are clay-coloured and constipated, or there may be a loose, bright yellow stool. The urine is dark yellow or brown from the bile pigments present. The chest may be affected with an irritating dry cough, or a sensation of dust in the throat, which may, when severe, develop into a right-sided bronchial pneumonia. Rheumatism affects the right hip, foot and ankle with swelling, tenderness and stiffness. Right-sided sciatica. The neck is stiff.

Modalities:

Better for: Eating, rest, cold drinks.

Worse for: Heat.

The China Constitution

Mentals:

Irritable, over-sensitive, adverse to being touched or looked at. Dull confusion, suicidal anxiety, weakness, fatigue, delirium.

General Indications for China as a remedy:

Collapse, exhaustion from loss of fluids.

Site of Action:

The body generally, although there is a particularly strong action on the gastro-intestinal tract, liver, spleen and lungs.

Symptoms:

Exhaustion, weakness, fatigue as in convalescence from loss of fluids, as in repeated haemorrhage from the uterus, lungs, bowels or nose. Excess lactation, sweating, mental or physical strain over a prolonged period of time can be causative factors. There is pallor, chill, sweating and coldness, face and cheeks sunken, the eyes encircled with dark rings. Headache is marked, throbbing and beating. The whole scalp is hyper-sensitive. Intermittent periodic fever may be present on alternate days with a sensation of burning heat after a chill.

The spleen is enlarged and tender, the liver sensitive, painful, with obstructing jaundice and a pale stool, the urine dark. Loss of sight and hearing with tinnitus. There is a bitter taste in the mouth, the tongue coated and dirty yellow. Flatulence of the whole abdomen is marked, with belching and rumbling abdominal noises. The appetite is impaired and they are indifferent to food although at times the opposite may occur with a voracious appetite. *China* feels full after the least food and generally digestion is slow and impaired. Gallstone colic may occur, there is characteristic painless diarrhoea – passing a watery stool, yellow, containing undigested faeces. Menorrhagia and leucorrhea are worse before a period. Haemorrhage may occur. The chest is affected with asthma, wheezy breathing, pneumonia, and there is profuse sweating, the whole skin chilly and hyper-sensitive to the least touch or draught. The *China* patient is usually thirsty. The extremities are often swollen and oedematous, and the lower limbs may feel cramped or numb.

Modalities:

Better for: Pressure, warmth.

Worse for: Touch, cold air, motion, midnight, eating fruit.

The Cimicifuga Constitution

Mentals:

Depressed, anxious, with frequent sighing, talking incessantly and disjointedly, restless. Everywhere is gloom and dejection, mental excitement, puerperal mania, psychosis. There is nervous tremor and shuddering.

General Indication for Cimicifuga as a remedy:

Uterine problems during pregnancy, menstrual difficulties, rheumatic problems of the low back.

Site of Action:

The mind and central nervous system, gastrointestinal tract, uterus and ovaries, chest, heart, lumbo-sacral region.

Symptoms:

Pain in the uterus and left ovary, with tenderness and a heavy sensation. Periods are irregular, painful, with cramping, labour-like pains, leucorrhea, nausea of pregnancy. *Cimicifuga* has a tonic action on the uterus, and makes labour easier. It is indicated where a previous foetus was still-born. There is headache, frontal or occipital, the head feels full and aching, with a pressure sensation pushing up the top of the skull and relieved by local pressure, worse but for movement. Epilepsy may be associated. The eyes are painful, the inhaled breath feels cold to the skull and brain. Facial neuralgia, particularly of the cheek, is common. The gastro-intestinal system is weak and upset with a coated tongue, foul breath and sinking sensation in the upper abdomen. There may be a dry, irritating cough, worse at night and from talking. Rheumatism, aching, sore, cramping pains especially of the left side of chest and neck, a feeling of weight in the lumbo-sacral area, and severe drawing pains in the upper thoracic vertebrae are often present. There may also be rheumatic chorea. There is a feeling of contraction, and pain is referred along the front of both thighs. The remedy is a very acute one, due to cold, damp, wet weather. Often opposite sides of the body are affected as left shoulder and right knee.

Modalities:

Better for: Warmth, eating.

Worse for: Night, windy damp weather, cold, movement.

The Cocculus Constitution

Mentals:

Timid, frightened, anxious, confused, sad, with-drawn, silent. There is hypersensitivity to noise and touch, with excessive over-reaction to anger or fear, sometimes grief. *Cocculus* is hypochondriacal, nervous, slow and apathetic. Time passes too quickly, fatigue is marked.

General Indications for Cocculus as a remedy:

Vertigo, nausea, vomiting, particularly from travel, paralytic weakness of muscles, abdominal colic and distension, usually mild, fair-haired people.

Site of Action:

Central nervous system, balance centres, voluntary muscles, and the gastro-intestinal tract.

Symptoms:

These are predominantly the symptoms of motion sickness with spinning dizziness and vertigo, nausea and vomiting. Headache, fatigue, with an empty floating sensation are associated. Slowness and apathy is marked, with weakness particularly of legs, hands and feet, trembling, giving way, hardly able to stand, the leg muscles lacking tone, and sensitive to touch. Liver is enlarged as also the abdomen which is distended, painful, with wind, colic, and loss of appetite. There is a metallic taste in the mouth and thirst for cold drinks. The windy colic and griping pains are worse at night (midnight) as also the painful periods, which have similar pains and occur every three weeks. Trembling and paralysis are common, with loss of sensation in hands and feet, weak legs, back and neck muscles. The head feels heavy. Hernia may develop.

Modalities:

Better for: Lying down quietly, sitting.

Worse for: Touch, jarring, movement, travel, eating or the smell of food, heat, the sun.

The Colchicum Constitution

Mentals:

Irritability, over-sensitivity, combined with a lethargy, slowness of mind and thought processes. Absence of fear or anxiety. Weakness and apathy are marked. *Colchicum* dislikes being touched or stroked, and is disinclined to move.

General Indications for Colchicum as a remedy:

Gout, rheumatism, severe diarrhoea with weakness and collapse as in typhoid fever.

Site of Action:

Colchicum acts on small joints of hands and feet mainly, affecting tendons, ligaments, periosteum, synovial membranes and muscles in the area affected. There is an acute inflammatory condition of the intestine affecting the mucous membrane. Heart and circulations, kidneys and urinary system are also affected.

Symptoms:

Severe, sudden gouty drawing, shifting, changeable pains in the small joints, especially toes and fingers, also wrists, which are swollen, stiff, dark red and hot, weak with a bruised, paralysed feeling.The grip is weak, and there is characteristic tingling in the finger nails. Pains are so severe that the patient may scream out. The body is generally cold, especially the legs and abdomen. Perspiration is marked, contrasting at the same time with periodic violent burning sensation, convulsions, cramps in the stomach and the abdomen and swollen intestines. There is a severe rice-water diarrhoea, with colic, urgency, and rectal spasm. The patient passes jelly-like mucous in the stool and numerous minute white flakes of shredded mucous membrane which may contain blood. Typhoid fever may be associated. The urine is dark, full of casts and albumin and has a heavy yellow deposit of uric acid. Weakness, slowness is everywhere and lack of strength, the head falling down on the chest, or the arms flop down by the side of the body. A peculiar symptom is that the left pupil may be tightly contracted, and the right widely dilated. There is hypersensitivity to cooking and kitchen smells especially of fish, even the thought may provoke nausea, weakness, to the point of fainting. The heart may be involved at times in the rheumatic process with palpitations, weakness, collapse, pericarditis and rarely the muscles of the ocular iris are also affected by the acute rheumatic process.

Modalities:

Better for: Rest, lying down, from bending forward.

Worse for: Motion, getting wet, chill, touch,
change to damp weather, in the
autumn, at night, from the smell of
cooking.

The Colocynth Constitution

Mentals:

Irritable, anxious, impatient, easily angered and offended by trifles. Morose and silent, unresponsive. Indignation is marked, grief, reluctance to talk.

General Indications for Colocynth as a remedy:

Severe doubling-up colic, diarrhoea, urinary frequency, arthritis of the large joints.

Site of Action:

Mainly affects the smooth involuntary muscle of the gastro-intestinal tract, genito-urinary system, and large joints of hip and low back.

Symptoms:

Severe pain is the major symptom. Colic, gripping cutting pains, agonising, twisting, constricting and doubling up, usually in the umbilical region and immediately after meals. The face is pale, cheeks drawn, and cold from anxiety. Dysentry and cholera may be present. There is jelly-like, watery diarrhoea, the urinary tract affected with frequency of urination and urgency passing a painful, scanty urine, of jelly-like clear consistency. Diarrhoea may be precipitated by indigestion, grief or anger, as also sudden amenorrhoea. Diabetes is sometimes associated. In the uterus and vagina, there may be dragging-down pains, with burning, tearing discomfort in the body generally. Gouty headaches, facial neuralgia, also involving the eye and eyeball. The large joints of the hip are affected and lumbo-sacral area with sciatic pain referred to the knee.

Modalities:

Better for: Passing flatus or stool, firm hand, local pressure, coffee, heat, warmth, doubling-up lying with head bent forward.

Worse for: Anger, indigestion, draught of cold air, movement, touch, eating fruit, at night.

The Conium Constitution

Mentals:

Depression, anxiety, tension, hypochondriasis, sexual problems, especially premature-ejaculation. Easily excitable. Memory is poor.

General Indications for Conium as a remedy:

Light-haired, often energetic elderly people with swelling in glandular tissue, as the breast, usually after a fall, blow or injury. Giddiness and urinary problems are often associated.

Site of Action:

Conium acts primarily on the lymphatic glandular tissues, and also affects the bladder, gastro-intestinal tract, genital organs, and central nervous system.

Symptoms:

There is a hardness of glandular tissues, particularly of the breast with sub-acute inflammation, following a blow, fall, or accident, sometimes with hardness and ulceration of overlying tissues. The breasts are tender and painful the day before or during a period, with stick-like pains, worse for jarring or movement. The testicles may be hard, swollen and bruised as from injury. Dizziness, vertigo and giddiness of the elderly is a feature, with a staggering, unsteady walk, always worsened by sudden head movements and change of position – as of suddenly turning the head, even moving the eyes, lying down or turning over. The eyes are also affected with a severe sensation of weakness, including drooping of the lids (ptosis) and corneal ulceration. General weakness and fainting is a feature, with an ascending paralysis, tremor, and stabbing rheumatic pain in the left hip. The genito-urinary system may be affected with sexual weakness, impotency and frequent interruption of the urine flow which is intermittent, stops and starts again, often associated with prostatic disorders of elderly men. Periods are weak and scanty. Flatulence and constipation are common, with nausea, heartburn – sometimes of pregnancy, and a burning sensation in the rectum. *Conium* has severe characteristic sweating on sleeping at anytime of the day or night. There is a dry, irritating cough, with laryngeal irritation. Constantly coughing or clearing the throat, the cough is usually worsened by lying down.

Modalities:

Better for: The dark, walking, movement, stooping, warmth, local pressure.

Worse for: Eating, standing, open air, bright light, touch, jar, fall.

The Cuprum Met Constitution

Mentals:

Restless, irritable, talkative, often impulsive with destructive wishes to injure others. Anger and fright are common. There may be confusion or delirium with much twitching and jerking. They are usually exhausted, mentally as well as physically.

General Indications for Cuprum met as a remedy:

Spasm is the principle indication, with cramps or convulsions. The spasm may involve the bronchial muscles with asthma, intestines with colic, uterus with dysmenorrhoea. They are usually fair-haired people.

Site of Action:

Mainly the smooth involuntary muscle of the body, and central nervous system.

Symptoms:

Cuprum has spasm and cramps as its main characteristic, with convulsions, restlessness, excitement, and irritability of the nervous system generally. Chorea, epilepsy, convulsions, may be present, with slowness of speech and clumsy, heavy, slow movements. The convulsive fits usually begin in the small muscles of the foot and then spread to involve the whole body. The tongue feels heavy and has a metallic taste, furred and dry with white coating and red edge to it. Stabbing pains are characteristic – as in the headaches, which are relieved by wrapping the head up.

Vomiting and hiccough may occur, the abdomen tense and hot with violent intermittent colic and severe cramping pains. Cholera. There is exhaustion, prostration and weakness, dysmenorrhoea is cramping and spasmodic, like all *Cuprum* pains. Asthma is often severe, the face red, lips and cheeks blue, with typical clutching of thumb and fingers as the spasm worsens. Usually they sit up in bed, unable to breathe deeply, thirsty for cold water. Coughing is violent, spasmodic and exhaustive, followed by palpitations, or suppression of breathing for a few seconds. The phlegm is whitish, the chest rattling with mucous. There may be laryngitis or croup.

Modalities:

Better for: Cold water drinks, wrapping the head up, sitting up.

Worse for: Before the menstrual period, walking quickly and effort, cold air, new moon, at night, cold wind.

287

The Drosera Constitution

Mentals:

Anxiety, depression, restlessness, pessimism, hypochondriasis.

General Indications for Drosera as a remedy:

Paroxysms of coughing with vomiting, whooping cough, often in children or the elderly.

Site of Action:

Inflammation of larynx and upper respiratory tract, joints, central nervous system, mucous membrane, involuntary muscle.

Symptoms:

There are attacks of dry hacking spasmodic coughing, which occur repeatedly and cause shortness of breath and difficulty in breathing. The paroxysms end in vomiting and retching – coughing up yellow mucous. The throat is sore and rough, the chest feels oppressed, and generally a child is pale, thin, with weak appetite and underweight. Hoarseness may be present, or an irritating sensation in the back of the throat as if there is a crumb or feather tickling the area which cannot be relieved. Spasms of sharp constricting pains suddenly occur in the larynx, throat, chest wall, and abdomen which may also include the genital area. There may be bleeding with bright red blood from the mouth, nose, sputum, vomit or stool. The bed feels to hard and uncomfortable. Pains in the hip joint, drawing or shooting. Sciatica may be suffered. Stitching pain in the shin moving down to the ankle. Cannot get comfortable. Shivery at rest, usually have night sweats, and swollen lymph glands somewhere in the body. Whooping cough, chronic tuberculosis and epilepsy are associated diseases.

Modalities:

Better for: Walking, movement, open air.

Worse for: The evening and after midnight, warmth or warm drinks, rest, lying in bed, talking.

The Dulcamara Constitution

Mentals:

Restless agitation, impatient and quarrelsome, critical without much overt anger.

General Indications for Dulcamara as a remedy:

Symptoms are always caused by cold and damp weather often following a change suddenly in the late summer weather, with hot days and cool nights. All problems are typically worse for cold and damp weather.

Site of Action:

Voluntary or involuntary muscles of the tongue, face, bladder, limbs, joints, gastro-intestinal tract, chest and skin. The central nervous system is also affected.

Symptoms:

Paralysis of the face as in Bells's Palsy, from a cold, damp draught of air, paralysis of the tongue as in motor neurone disease, cerebral or throat tumours. Bladder or limbs may be paralysed, also heart or lungs but always aggravated or precipitated by exposure to cold and damp, or a change of weather. The paralysed parts and extremities are icy cold. There may be symptoms of excitation of the nervous system with spasm, tremor, convulsions and shaking. Griping abdominal pains are common, with colic and a yellow, watery stool, sometimes vomiting after the motion is passed. There is an offensive sweat, the skin is unhealthy, covered with a red damp nettle-rash urticarian eruption, with itching and irritation, which may also involve the tongue. There may be warts or skin ulcers, particularly of the face. Catarrh is common, with upper respiratory tract infection which may develop into bronchitis with cough and blood-stained sputum, or asthma with a loose rattling moist cough. Pain in the neck and low back from catching cold with tearing, shooting, drawing pains radiating down both thighs and associated soreness. There may be rheumatic paralysis of the legs with swelling, oedema, weakness but especially icy coldness. Any change of weather worsens the symptoms when atmospheric pressure falls.

Modalities:

Better for: Movement, warmth, walking erect posture, dry weather.

Worse for: Cold or damp weather, rest, stooping, bending, cold air, cold drinks, ice cream, getting wet or damp, in the afternoon and evening, sudden changes of weather.

The Ferrum Metallicum Constitution

Mentals:

There is excessive sensitivity and irritability, especially to noises, which are felt to be unbearable. Restless, weak, depressed and quarrelsome, reluctant to talk. Anorexia Nervosa.

General Indications for Ferrum met. as a remedy:

Anaemia, weakness, often with associated digestive upsets, or chest symptoms.

Site of Action:

Blood and circulation, gastro-intestinal tract, lung, uterus and bladder.

Symptoms:

Weakness, fatigue, pallor, chill, breathless and fainting. Anaemia of young people, with a pale, greenish face and mucous membrane. The cheeks may also be red and flushed worse from the least effort and with sudden flushes of heat to face and head. There is frequently a pulsating, hammer-like headache, and throbbing pains in the limbs and body. Facial neuralgia. Cramps. Haemorrhages are common, the pulse full, yielding to pressure. Blood is lost from the nose, uterus, lungs, kidney, stomach. Feet and ankles are frequently swollen.

The genito-urinary system is affected with either absent periods, particularly in delicate, young anorexic girls, or more commonly they are too early, heavy, the flow prolonged. Impotence, sterility, miscarriage may occur, the vagina is dry. They may be constipated, more common is a painless diarrhoea after eating or drinking after midnight. The stool is undigested. Incontinence of urine on standing, the abdomen tender and sore and there is nausea, flatulence, vomiting, loss of appetite alternating with bouts of compulsive eating. Regurgitation of food. Vertigo and dizziness on rising. Asthma, cough, breathing laboured and difficult, worse for the slightest effort. Rheumatism of large joints especially left shoulder and upper arm, with paralysing, tearing, shooting, pains, so that raising the arm is impossible. Lumbago. They often get up at night and walk about slowly for relief.

Modalities:

Better for: Slow walking and movement, warmth.

Worse for: After midnight, cold, quick movement, eggs, meat, eating or drinking.

The Gelsemium Constitution

Mentals:

Fearful, anxious, nervous, over-sensitive, tends to be hysterical and dramatic. Anxiety is anticipatory, with stage-fright and examination nerves. Usually they are quiet and still, want to be left alone, sleepy and dull, cannot gather thoughts, and may be weepy or suicidal. There is a fear of falling, yet impulses to throw themselves from a height. Hysterical lump in the throat, impotence.

General Indications for Gelsemium as a remedy:

Weakness, prostration, paralysis and tremor. Indicated for nervous young people and children of hysterical make-up.

Site of Action:

Mainly the nervous supply to voluntary muscles, mind and central nervous system.

Symptoms:

Paralysis with weakness and tremor is characteristic. Eyelids droop and internal eye muscles are paralysed leading to double vision, blurring of the vision. The tongue is numb and thick, the oesophagus weak with swallowing difficulties and the anus may be open and lacking tone, with a yellowish diarrhoea – often of nervous origin, from emotion or anticipation. Dizziness and vertigo are marked and there is dull headache, beginning at the back of the head and moving forward over the whole head. Dilated pupils, the headache relieved by passing urine and aggravated by any delay in passing urine.

Typhoid fever, paralysis after diptheria, measles, writer's cramp, convulsion, epilepsy, coryza, 'flu', hay fever, a flushed face, early morning sneezing, and a streaming cold. Chills up and down the spine, muscles of the back tender. The uterus is full and feels heavy, periods cramp-like and paralysed. *Gelsemium* is usually restless. The heart is often weak, the pulse soft and irregular. A useful remedy in glaucoma.

Modalities:

Better for: Local heat, cool days and fresh air.

Worse for: Movement, damp, fog, sudden changes in weather, thunder.

The Glonoine Constitution

Mentals:

Anxious, agitated, depressed and fearful. Depression, delirium, comatosed. They lose their way in familiar surroundings due to the confusional state.

General Indications for Glonoine as a remedy:

Headache following exposure to heat or from fear or shock. Sunstroke from exposure to excessive direct or indirect heat.

Site of Action:

Central nervous system and circulation.

Symptoms:

Violent, bursting, explosive headaches. Sudden pain of acute, rapid onset. Throbbing, violent, stabbing and expansive neuralgic pains, often felt to begin in the neck, spreading to temples, forehead and whole head. Neuralgic pains worse from any movement or jarring. There is a rush of blood to the head and flashes of heat to the heart and chest. Heat stroke. Sunstroke. Vertigo worse on standing or rising. The face is flushed, menopausal flushes. Fainting, loss of consciousness, nausea and vomiting. Epilepsy, convulsions, especially of labour. The chin feels long, lower lip swollen. The least pressure on the head causes worsening of the head pains. Generally the head also feels too large and there is a feeling of throbbing fullness. Angina pectoris.

Modalities:

Better for: Open air, rest, cool applications.

Worse for: At night, for head-jarring, bright lights, warmth.

The Graphites Constitution

Mentals:

Sad, anxious, depressed, weeping easily. Fearful, changeable with mood swings. Pessimistic, reluctant to work, music causes weeping.

General Indications for Graphites as a remedy:

Graphites is fair, chilly, always cold and exhausted generally, with marked skin problems which ooze. Disturbances of digestion and involving the whole body.

Site of Action:

Skin, gastro-intestinal tract, lymphatic system, circulation, joints, genito-urinary system, mind.

Symptoms:

There is chronic eczema, with rough, dry, cracked skin, scaly, itchy, red, sweating and irritating, which oozes a thick sticky glutinous honey-coloured fluid. Particularly on the face and behind the ears, but also involving the scalp and eyelids, which are fissured and covered with crusts and scabs. Lips, mouth, nostrils and anus are cracked and a moist eczema may involve the feet or genito-anal area. There is a cobweb-like sensation on the face. *Graphites* is always chilly -inside or out of doors, drowsy, yawning, tired, the eyelids heavy. There is weakness of the whole body with exhaustion and prostration. Vertigo is common with a full intoxicated feeling in the head. Eyes are red and eczematous, watering easily and flicker. Photophobia. There is a heavy weight-like headache, mainly of the occipital region. Lymph glands are often swollen, tender and enlarged due to secondary infection of the eczema. Cheeks are red and flushed. Hot flushes with a rush of blood to the face. Faintness. Slowness is common, the whole body and tissues generally relaxed. The stools are frequently either constipated, pale, covered with mucous, or thin, watery and offensive, containing undigested particles. Periods are usually either absent or delayed. The breasts are painful at period time when itching in the genito-anal area is aggravated. Distention of upper abdomen is a feature with poor appetite. Flatulence and colicky cramping pains, better for eating. The tongue is clean, often ulcerated on the underside or tip. Nose bleeds are common. Deafness is often helped. Impotence. Leucorrhoea – with a profuse white mucous discharge. Finger nails are thickened and tend to grow out of shape. *Graphites* removes induration from old scars. Useful in styes. Rheumatism of the neck. Sweat is offensive, worse at night, and stains clothes yellow. Urine is thick with a white deposit.

Modalities:

Better for: Rest, eating, warm drinks.

Worse for: Movement, and exertion, cold
drinks, cold air, warmth of bed
aggravates the itching, Summer
and Autumn, sweet food, meat or
fish, music.

The Hepar Sulph Constitution

Mentals:

Irritable, impetuous, easily cross, takes offence, angry and abusive with passionate impulses to kill, burn or destroy. Dissatisfied with self, dreamy and preoccupied. Sadness, dejection to the point of becoming suicidal. They are very nervous and start fearfully when sleeping.

General Indications for Hepar sulph as a remedy:

Chilly, over-sensitive people, with acute inflammation of throat, skin, or chest, with a tendency to abcess formation and purulent discharges. Usually they are fair-haired and slow, overweight.

Site of Action:

Lymphatic system, skin, mucous membrane of the respiratory tract.

Symptoms:

The key symptom is hypersensitivity to any external stimulus – which causes an aggravation. Dry, cold air, noise, odours, a draught, the slightest touch or pressure worsens the condition. The least pain may result in an over-reaction such as fainting. The *Hepar* patient takes cold quickly, and must be covered. The throat is frequently affected with a cold, soreness, and splinter-like or fish-bone sensations with a sticking feeling on swallowing and pain in the ears.

There may be quinsy with absess formation of the tonsil area, and throbbing, stabbing pain. The nose is swollen and sore to touch, catarrh is marked. Coughing and shortness of breath may occur, the cough may become worse on un-covering. Headache, bronchitis, pneumonia and asthma. Rigors, fever, sweating day and night. Mastoid abcess and chronic inflam-matory problems.

The skin is unhealthy with a nettle-rash like eruption, unhealthy ulcers which suppurate and discharge, with moist soreness in the genito-anal area. The ulcers bleed at the slightest touch. Itching is marked. Inflam-mation of the throat, sometimes also involving the chest, bowels or kidneys. Constipation is a feature with an absence of power to expel a soft, clay-coloured sour-smelling and offensive stool. Much urging is needed. The bladder is weak, with delay, the flow weak, slow to pass and finish. Sweating is marked, particularly at night.

Modalities:

Better for: Warm wet weather, acid foods, fats, vinegar, wrapping up.

Worse for: Dry, cold weather, cold appli-cations, lying on painful side.

The Hypericum Constitution

Mentals:

Nervous depression, shock, fright after wounds.

General Indications for Hypericum as a remedy:

Pain, haemorrhage, tenderness whenever there has been damage to nervous tissue and nerve endings, particularly by a puncture wound.

Site of Action:

The body generally, but particularly areas of the body that are richly innervated such as the tips of the fingers, spine and coccyx.

Symptoms:

Tearing, stitching, needle-like pains, sharp, with paralytic weakness of the affected part. Particularly indicated in puncture wounds as from pin or nail, splinter or bite. There is tenderness and ulcerations of the wound. Bunions and corns. The abdomen distended with cutting-like pains. Pains after abdominal surgery. Concussion. Acute labour pains. Asthma, with tightness of the chest, pneumonia. Whooping cough, palpitations, bleeding piles.

Modalities:

Better for: Rest, quiet, lying on the affected
side.

Worse for: Cold, damp air, fog, touch,
draughts.

The Ignatia Constitution

Mentals:

Sudden mood changes, rapidly with sobbing, sighing, grief, gaiety, weeping, depression. Hopeless, wants to be alone, easily moved to anger, quarrelsome and impatient. Conscientious. Hysterical. Delusional. Silent suppressed grieving. Sensitive, too easily impressionable, worse from fright.

General Indications for Ignatia as a remedy:

Indicated whenever there is the typical *Ignatia* mentality, with sudden acute paroxysmal, changeable symptoms elsewhere in the body, often spasmodic in type.

Site of Action:

Mainly affects the mind, central nervous system, gastro-intestinal tract, genito-urinary system.

Symptoms:

Spasm with nervous twitching, facial tics, convulsions, the face pale. Pains are severe, often excessive, varying in character, headache worse for tobacco smoke, and relieved by passing urine. Sore throat better for swallowing food, tonsillitis, diphtheria. Hysterical sensation of a lump or ball in the throat.

Headaches – as a nail driven through the skull. Eyes inflamed and photophobia, weakness in the pit of stomach. Food may be regurgitated, with hiccough, hysterical vomiting, loss of voice. Like the sore throat, toothache is better for eating. There is a dry, hoarse, hacking cough. Periods are painful, with bearing-down pains, in the abdomen, the flow black, offensive with clots. Sourness is a feature with a sour taste in the mouth. Piles, rectal prolapse, anal spasms, sharp burning pains in the rectum and anus. There is great urgency. Constipation. The limbs jerk on falling asleep. Chorea. Epilepsy. Intermittent fever with thirst only present at the stage of feeling chilly, but not otherwise.

Modalities:

Better for: Lying on painful side, swallowing solids, passing urine.

Worse for: Anger, anxiety, tobacco smoke.

The Ipecacuanha Constitution

Mentals:

Depressed, irritable, vague, impatient, nothing pleases, disinclined to talk or work, cannot endure the least noise. Anxious, fear of suffocation.

General Indications for Ipecacuanha as a remedy:

Constant unrelieved nausea and vomiting, haemorrhage, chest and gastro-intestinal symptoms.

Site of Action:

Gastro-intestinal tract, circulations. Especially affects the mucous membrane of the respiratory and genito-urinary tracts.

Symptoms:

Constant nausea is the predominant and key symptom, unrelieved by vomiting. There is a profuse, excessive salivation, which is frequently swallowed, tongue clean, the stomach feeling relaxed, empty and hanging down. There may be vomiting of mucous, bile or bright red blood. The face is pale green, drawn, the mouth curled down, eyes dark-ringed. Bleeding is common, from anywhere in the body, particularly nose, throat, mouth, also lungs, bowels, and uterus. Nausea is associated with the haemorrhage.

Menorrhagia is common, or threatened abortion with abdominal pains radiating from navel downwards to the uterus. Bleeding may occur after a confinement, and is profuse and constant. Periods are excessive and too early. Vaginal irritation, leucorrhoea (thick discharge) labour is usually weak. Fibroids. Headache is common, bruised in character either due to indigestion or rheumatism. Diarrhoea is a feature with the passage of green, foamy fermented stools associated with colicky pains and nausea. There is loud, noisy, rattling breathing heard all over the room. Cough is dry with suffocating spasmodic shortness of breath, gasping, vomiting and wheezing asthma a sensation of weight in the chest. The child is blue, rigid and stiff. Pneumonia. Emphysema of the elderly. Disgust for food. Intermittent fevers. Backache. The extremities are cold and pespiring. The eyes are affected with conjuntivitis, lids granulated. Neuralgic pains, subacute corneal inflammation, photophobia.

Modalities:

Better for: Cold drinks, rest, closing eyes, local pressure.

Worse for: Touch, movement, winter, dry weather, rich food – as pork, eating, morning and evening 6-7 p.m.

The Lachesis Constitution

Mentals:

Thin, sad, despondent, irritable. Anxiety and depression with feelings of insecurity, jealousy, hatred, suspicion, envy. Cruelty, conceit and self-consiousness. Confusion is common with mistakes in writing, poor memory, and a disturbed sense of time. They are also over-active, talk excessively, become confused, manic with delirium, fever.

General Indications for Lachesis as a remedy:

The typical *Lachesis* patient is often female, of irritable disposition, with red hair and freckles. Left-sided pain, severe inflammation of the body particularly involving throat and mind. Worse for sleep and any constriction in the area. There is purple discolouration of the part affected.

Site of Action:

The body generally, particularly throat, gastro-intestinal tract, lungs, circulation, genito-urinary system and skin.

Symptoms:

Thin, weak, exhausted, the symptoms are nearly always left-sided and worse for sleep. *Lachesis* is a night owl and always feels worse in the morning. The whole body is affected with headache over the eyes and root of the nose. Tinnitus and vertigo on waking or closing eyes, the sight dim with flickering sensations in the field of vision. Tremor is marked, of hands and body generally, the tongue dry, shaking and catches in the teeth. There is loss of appetite. *Lachesis* is often alcoholic and there is the typical red nose of the spirit drinker. Fainting, convulsions, spasm.

Haemorrhage is a feature and small wounds bleed profusely, the blood dark, and may be decomposed. Infection, with boils, carbuncles, bed sores, malaria, malignant scarlet fever, diptheria, smallpox, appendicitis, pneumonia, typhoid fever, plague, the overlying skin area is blue, blackish, purple. The throat is strongly affected with an ulcerated sore throat, left face and jaw swollen, worse from bending the head back, for touch or pressure of clothes. Sensation of a lump, crumb or fish-bone in the throat. Pain is left-sided and felt in the left ear. Toothache worse on waking, after eating, and from warm drinks. The liver and spleen may be tender, swollen, sore, and engorged. There is a characteristic sensation of a 'ball' or lump in the throat, bladder abdomen or rectum of a 'plug' in the anal region. Urine is dark, foaming with blackspots, and night-time frequency. Diarrhoea with a dark offensive stools, like charred wheat-straw, followed by burning, throbbing pain in the anus. Haemorrhoids are burning with a stitch-like pains and anal spasm. Painful swelling of the left ovary.

Periods are scanty, painful just before the flow, but regular until the menopause, with hot-flushes, sweating, burning headaches, flooding. Breasts are swollen, painful with swelling of the left breast from infection, abcess or tumour. There is a dry hacking, tickling cough, short-ness of breath, asthma. The least tightness of clothes on the chest or neck is intolerable. Cramp-like pains. Palpitations, anxiety, an-gina pectoris. Blueness, cyanosis, varicose veins. Burning, scalding pains in the body generally as from a severe burn. Weakness and exhaustion physically and mentally is seen. Shingles.

Modalities:

Better for: Cold applications, eating, fruit, open air, rest.

Worse for: Spring, mild cloudy weather, sleep, tight constrictive clothes, sun, draughts, hot drinks, in the morn-ing and on waking, from move-ment.

The Magnesia Carbonica Constitution

Mentals:

Anxious, fearful, exhausted. Irritable, nervous, sad, sensitive, indisposed to talk. Symptoms follow a severe shock or emotional stress.

General Indications for Mag carb as a remedy:

Fatigue, exhaustion, with diarrhoea and griping pains.

Site of Action:

Gastro-intestinal tract, reproductive system, joints of upper arm.

Symptoms:

Exhaustion, fatigue, worn-out, particularly indicated in women after childbirth or prolonged strain. Neuralgic pains, usually left-sided with shooting pains in the face, gums and orbit. Pyorrhoea. Nausea and toothache of pregnancy. Abdomen is distended, and there is vomiting with a thin, watery green or blood-stained stool. Colic and griping pains. Thirst and sweating is marked. The *Mag carb* child is thin, small, weak, undersized, refusing milk, with the typical greenish stool. The face is drawn and thin, the eyes have dark rings.

Sourness is characteristic. Stools, sweat, breath, vomit, taste is sour. Periods are painful with colic and backache, flowing only at night, when lying down, and stopping on walking. The flow is dark, thick and excoriating. Rheumatism of arm and shoulder is a feature, pain worse on raising arm with weakness. Wrist, finger and knees may be involved, with cramps in the calves at night. Intolerant of heat, they feel too hot in bed, and throw off the covers. Severe rheumatic pain at rest.

Modalities:

Better for: Cool room.

Worse for: Night, heat, turning in bed,
                    2-3.00 a.m.

The Magnesium Phosphorica Constitution

Mentals:

Nervous, hypochondriacal, depressed and anxious, often forgetful, drowsy, unable to concentrate.

General Indications for Mag. phos. as a remedy:

Thin, dark-complexioned people. Acute neuralgia or colic, cramps, spasm.

Site of Action:

Muscles of the body generally, particularly intestines and uterus.

Symptoms:

Severe cramping, neuralgic, stabbing pains, boring and constricting. Pains are shifting which come and go. Cramps, toothache, writer's cramp, headache. Cramps of stomach, around the umbilicus. Spasms in whooping cough, tetanus, chorea. Hiccough, cramp and spasm of the calf muscle. Usually it is a right-sided remedy. A useful remedy in dysmennorrhoea cramping pains during a period cause doubling-up with violent spasms. Headache.

Modalities:

Better for: Heat, pressure, warmth, hot drinks, bending double when the cramps occur.

Worse for: Cold air or cold water. Uncovering, light touch, at night.

The Mercurius Constitution

Mentals:

Weakness of mind, changeable, restless, quick speech and thoughts. Everything is precipitate and hurried, yet there is weak memory, and will, depression, no desire to live. Agitation, excitable, anxious, delirium, hallucinations. Time passes slowly, vague and absent-minded.

General Indications for Mercurius as a remedy:

Acute infection of the body generally with a tendency to abcess formation. Profuse offensive sweating. Chill, weakness, intolerant of heat.

Site of Actions:

The body generally, especially skin, throat, gastro-intestinal, respiratory and genito-urinary tracts.

Symptoms:

There is a foul, offensive breath which has a peculiar sweetish and mercurial odour, with profuse perspiration, drenching the body with yellow, offensive, oily sweat, day and night. The whole body is weak, exhausted and rest-less. Creeping chilliness with tendency to fainting, particularly after a bowel motion. Thirst is marked and persistent – for cold drinks. There is a sweetish, slimy, metallic taste, the mouth full of saliva which is constantly swallowed. *Mercurius* tongue is moist, has a whitish coating, feels thick and flabby, has teeth imprints on the sides. Hands and feet are cold, covered with chilly profuse sweat yet intolerant of warmth or cold and worse for the heat of the bed.

Inflammation and infection is marked with ulcer and abcess formation and pus. Gums are swollen, spongy, bleeding easily. Tonsils are red with a stitch-like pain referred to the ear, and enlarged with a purulent discharge. The nose is red. Catarrh, burning, excoriating and dirty looking. Oedema and discharges are offensive. Nosebleeds in sleep. Ears are inflamed and there may be a yellow blood-stained discharge from the right ear with tearing pains. The face is drawn, eyes dark ringed, drawn together, tired, with burning pains and infections. The mouth may be ulcerated at the corners. Severe pulsating toothache may occur, usually worse at night. There may be ulceration of the skin with a greasy, grey, pale-based ulcer, the sides red and raw, protruding outwards. Tremor is a feature of the body generally, and may involve the tongue, feet and hands. Usually it begins in the fingers. Parkinsonism, convulsions, epilepsy. Liver enlarged and tender, with stitch-like pains, and inability to lie on the right side. The gastrointestinal tract is affected with an exhausting, colicky diarrhoea. Stools are slimy, bloodstained and green, with urgency and burning constricting pains before and afterwards. There is a constant desire to urinate, but little is passed and there may be burning pains in the urethra. Profuse leucorrhoea, burning and itching, usually worse at night. Skin is infected with pustular eruptions, infected eczemous conditions, bleeding ulcers, which look moist, offensive and dirty. Shingles, smallpox, malignant scarlet fever and severe acute infection of the body generally as bronchitis, pneumonia, peri-tonitis. Lymph glands are infected and enlarged, without heat, like the rest of the body they are cold or covered with oily, offensive sweat. Inflammatory rheumatism of the joints, with tearing, shooting, drawing pains of the shoulders, arms, wrists and fingers. The patient is always chilly, asks for a hot water bottle, but quickly becomes overheated, throws off the covers, wants the window open and then rapidly becomes chilled again. They are very changeable.

Modalities:

Better for: Rest, lying down, in the morning.

Worse for: Night, warmth or cold, cold air or draughts, touch of pressure, meat, fats, coffee, lying on the right side.

The Phytolacca Constitution

Mentals:

Depressed, sad, indifferent to life, irritable. Over-sensitive people. Delirium, restless.

General Indications for Phytolacca as a remedy:

Severe sore throat, inflammatory conditions, tumours and inflammation of the breast.

Site of Action:

Phytolacca particularly affects the throat, breast tissues and joints.

Symptoms:

The throat is painful with acute shooting pains, hot, burning and dry, mucous membrane dark red, tonsils swollen with white spots. Pain is severe on swallowing and radiates into both ears. Diptheria. Vomiting. Diarrhoea may occur, and severe frontal headache, usually settling over the right eye. Pains are sharp, sudden, and move about, the phlegm tough, thick, offensive and stringy. The tip of the tongue is red, and on swallowing pain is felt in the root of the tongue. There is prostration, with fever. Lymph glands of the neck are swollen and tender. Pains in the breast are characteristic – with mastitis, tumour, abcess, pain in the nipple when nursing, the affected breast hard, full, swollen, hot and painful. Dysmennorrhoea. Spasm in the anal-rectal area with a blood discharge. Rheumatism may involve the whole body – with sudden unbearable shifting pains, shock-like and catching. Ankles are swollen, pains move from the outer limb area inwards. Sciatica is on the outer border of the leg. Lumbago. Inability to raise the right arm or shoulder, stiff neck, torticollis, obesity. Erythema Nodosum.

Modalities:

Better for: Heat of the bed, raising the heels higher than the head.

Worse for: Night, damp weather, movement on walking.

The Rhus Tox Constitution

Mentals:

Restless in mind and body, sad, weeps easily. Worries about business problems. Insomnia, weariness. The restless state of mind may become worse and confused with delirium.

General Indications for Rhus tox as a remedy:

Rheumatism and arthritic conditions of large and small joints of the body. Worse for rest, better for heat and continued movement. Urticarial and eczematous skin conditions.

Site of Action:

Rhus tox acts on muscular and fibrous tissues of the whole body, especially joints, skin, mucous membrane and lymphatic tissues.

Symptoms:

Pain, stiffness, paralysis and rigidity, worse from exposure to damp cold and better for warmth and activity. There is aching, bruised, sprained pain, tense and tingling, the muscles sore, with weakness and loss of strength. Rest and sleep aggravates, as when first getting out of bed or on a chair, but warmth, continued motions and exercise improve pain and stiffness. Pain and soreness is responsible for the restlessness at night and is a key characteristic of the remedy. Lumbago, sprains from strains and lifting, or over-stretching, sciatica.

The skin and mucous membrane is affected, eyes red, sore and inflamed, with conjuctivitis, lids swollen, stiff and heavy with a sticky discharge. Tongue is dry, with a red sore tip. The throat may be swollen and also lymphatic glands in the neck region, particularly the parotids and submaxillary glands. Urticaria, or eczema. Erysipelas, with a red itchy rash, inflamed and swollen with multiple transparent blisters and a slimy discharge. Thirst is marked, especially for milk, with dryness of throat. Cough, nausea – worse at rest. Vertigo is better for movement but worse on sitting. Rheumatism of the jaw. Nocturnal enuresis. Dysentery with tearing pains. Intermittent fevers. *Rhus* is always chilly, but craves cold drinks which worsen the symptoms. The cause is usually cold, getting wet, a chill or from damp.

Modalities:

Better for: Warmth, continued movement and exercise.

Worse for: Cold damp, rest or sitting, in the morning.

The Ruta Constitution

Mentals:

Anxious, irritable, depressed, tends to be mistrustful.

General Indications for Ruta as a remedy:

Bruised, arthritic, rheumatic pains of large joints, especially knees. The eyes are frequently affected.

Site of Action:

The periosteum, large joints, visual apparatus.

Symptoms:

Pain in the knees, tearing, burning and bruised which may involve hips and ankles. There is restlessness and weakness, the whole body uncomfortable on lying down, with constant efforts to get comfortable. Burning is present in the eyes which are heavy, tired and strained, with a weight-like sensation, often after excess reading. There may be fever with sweating and headache. Periods are usually weak or absent. Epilepsy. Facial paralysis.

Modalities:

Better for: Movement and rest, the backache is improved by lying down on the back.

Worse for: Cold, damp, touch, pressure.

PART THREE

Chapter Thirty-four

Guidelines to finding your own Constitutional Remedy

What follows attempts to clarify some of the multiple factors used in homoeopathy to assess a patient's 'constitutional' and to help the reader find his or hers. In the following pages the steps have been simplified to help with some of the problems of self-assessment and the limitations of this method.

No guarantee can be given that the following method will unerringly lead to your constitutional remedy. But I hope that in at least some cases it will be successful. It is not easy – even in the consulting room. I also hope that the following sheets will have some interest and value to the reader – if only to provoke the exercise of constitutional self-assessment. This may lead on to further thoughts and discussion as well as giving a greater understanding into the many factors concerned with its evaluation by the physician.

If you ask a physician to assess his or her own 'constitutional' they may have just as many problems as the reader. It is not easy, but try the exercises if only to see the intrinsic difficulties and you may also be able to improve on the present model, if your own constitutional remedy does not clearly emerge.

General Introduction to Finding Your Basic Constitutional Remedy

Rate yourself according to the five major areas of physiological and psychological functioning given, as accurately as possible for each of the areas listed.

1. Body Shape (Symbols 1-4), page 337

2. Energy Levels (Symbols A-E), page 338

3. The Weakest area of the Body where Illness Tends to Occur (Symbols Σ-Θ), page 339-341

4. The Modalitites, or Factors of Aggravation or Amelioration (Symbols page 342)

5. Basic Personality and Temperament (Symbols a-f) page 343-344

Write down the appropriate symbols given in the correct order to give you the constitutional coding which applies to you. In this way match your own personality and physiological profile with that of the nearest remedy. If this is not immediately clear, take the three nearest codings from the list which most closely match your own individual coding. Then read the detailed constitutional profiles of each in the clinical constitutional data sheets (chapters 32 & 33). Find the one that best fits you in overall totality in terms of temperament and physiological characteristics. The data sheet which gives you the closest 'fit' to yourself gives the constitutional remedy.

A Practical Example of Constitutional Coding.

Beginning with body shape, a very thin person would rate themselves as (1) from the descriptions and the codings which are given in brackets each time. The second consti-tutional point relates to energy-availability. Because they have energy to spare, they rate themself as D. from the description given. The third constitutional point is concerned with the most vulnerable area of the body. As they have a history of peptic ulcer and chronic problems of flatulence and indigestion the code (Θ) is chosen. The fourth point relates to the modalities or factors of aggravation or amelioration.

Because he feels better for a damp day, the symbol which reflects this –

is chosen.

The final constitutional point is based on temperament and personality. Easily short-tempered and often irritable, he chooses the irritable-impulsive coding group which gives the symbol (e).

This gives a final coding reading of .

1. D. Θ   e

Matched against the constitutional coding reference-sheet, the constitutional remedy is given as *Nux vomica*. The two nearest alternative choices, when the clinical data sheets are needed, are *Lachesis* or *Silicea*.

Body Shape

Thin and underweight (1)

Physique is definitely and severely underweight for individual height and bone structure.

Slimly built (2)

Physique is on the slim side but with no severe problems of weight-loss.

Average for height, weight and age (3)

Physique is satisfactory and well within normal expected limits for bone structure, age and height.

Roundly proportioned with a tendency to excess weight (4)

Moderately and evidently over-weight with the excess present as fat which rounds body shape but not excessively. Sometimes considerably over-weight.

Energy Levels

Exhausted with no energy reserves (A)

There is chronic exhaustion and fatigue with no strength or reserves. The least thing tires and adds to a sense of being worn-out.

Easily tired, particularly after period of effort (B)

Tired with no reserves or energy to spare after a reasonable effort or working day.

Energy levels good, but tired at the end of a working day (C)

There is enough energy for most of the daily work-load but nevertheless over-tired at the end of a normal working day.

Energy to spare, whatever the work-load (D)

Energised and with energy to spare whatever the working day has brought and whatever the chores.

Often in a 'high' over-active phase of energy surplus, unable to wind down. (E)

The energy level is over-charged to a degree of being in a 'high' most of the time, and over-active. Unable to relax or wind-down at the end of the day.

Your weakest, most vulnerable areas of the body where physical illness tends to occur and recur.

Skin, and Underlying Tissues (Σ)

This may commonly take the form of such problems as recurrent acne, itching of the skin, eczema, boils, psoriasis, cracking of the skin.

Digestive Organs (Θ)

Such symptoms as indigestion, wind, flatulence, heart-burn, pain after meals, loss of appetite, etc.

Circulation (Γ)

Chilblains, 'dead' fingers, hot-sweats, cold feet, blood pressure, etc.

Kidney and Bladder (Ξ)

Problems as renal colic, renal stones, pyelitis, recurrent cystitis, frequency, 'nervous' bladder, etc.

Bowel dysfunction (E)

The common problems are chronic constipation, chronic use of laxatives, diarrhoea, colitis, diverticulitis, rectal spasm, etc.

Liver and Gall Bladder (Π)

Typical problems are gall stones, gall stone colic, jaundice, hepatitis, generally liverish, intolerance of fats, etc.

Chest and Lungs (Ω)

Common symptoms are bronchitis, emphysema, recurrent colds, pneumonia, asthma, etc.

Heart (Z)

Shortness of breath, ankle-swelling, angina, heart attack, tachycardia, palpitations, dropped beats, rheumatic carditis, mitral stenosis, pacemaker, etc.

Joints (ψ)

Arthritis, rheumatism, swelling, stiffness, pain.

Central Nervous System (H)

Degeneration of muscles, nerves, weakness of speech, spasticity, lack of coordination, fits, 'blackouts'.

Reproductive System (Δ)

Discharge, prolapse, sexual problems, period difficulties, infection, miscarriage, problems of fertility.

Throat and Sinuses (O)

Recurrent sore throats, catarrh, and sinusitis, repeated colds and 'flu'.

Modalitites Or Factors Of Aggravation Or Improvement.

I generally feel	Better for	Worse for
Heat		
Cold		
Dryness		
Damp		

Basic Personality and Temperament.

Confident and outgoing (a)

Enjoys the company of others, able to be fairly confident and to relate socially in a reasonably relaxed easy manner.

Less confident, anxious (b)

Less sure in social situations, with a tendency to interpret body symptoms in a more pessimistic way.

Variability of mood (c)

Mood is rather variable from day to day with 'lows' on some days or pessimism but happy at other times, quickly changing again from laughter to tears.

Depressive-withdrawn (d)

The predominant mood is one of 'lows' of pessimism more consistently and frequently than in the above group. There is a lack of confidence and a greater tendency to avoid and withdraw from contact with others.

Irritable-impulsive (e)

At times there is a short fuse with a quick tendency to boil-over with easily provoked rage and anger which seemed justifiable at the time but later is regretted. Over-reaction and impulsiveness.

Phobic-dependent (f)

There are problems of panic and anxiety in certain situations with limited confidence or anxiety which can reduce activity and contacts, causing over- dependence.

Personal Constitutional Codings:

1	A	W		b	Arsenicum
1	A	Γ		b	Baryta carb
1	A	Θ		b	Carbo veg.
1	A	Θ		b	Mag.carb.
1	A	ψ		b	Rhus tox.
1	A	Θ		d	Mag.phos.
1	A	Γ		e	Ferrum met.
1	A	Σ		f	Silicea.
1	D	Θ		e	Nux vomica

1	E	Δ		d	Lachesis
2	A	Θ		b	Cocculus
2	A	H		c	Cuprum, met
2	A	Σ		d	Graphites
2	A	Δ		e	Sepia
2	A	Θ		e	Ipecacuanha
2	A	Θ		f	Argentum Nit.
2	B	Θ		b	Lysopodium
2	B	Ξ		b	Natrum mur.

2	B	Π		b	Phosphorus
2	C	Θ		e	Colycynth.
2	E	Γ		a	Agaricus
2	E	Θ		e	Chamomilla
2	E	Ξ		e	Cantharis
3	A	Σ		e	Thuja
3	A	Ω		e	Ammonium tart.
3	A	Θ		e	Aethusa
3	B	Δ		d	Cimifuga

3	B	H		d	Hypericum
3	B	Ξ		d	Benzoic ac
3	B	Ψ		e	Colchicum
3	B	Σ		f	Arnica
3	B	Ω		b	Drosera
3	D	H		d	Phytolacca
3	E	Σ		e	Belladonna
4	A	Π		b	Chelidonium
4	A	Σ		e	Bryonia

4	A	Π		e	China
4	A	Σ		f	Mercurius
4	A	H		f	Gelsemium
4	B	E		b	Alumina
4	B	Θ		b	Borax
4	B	Ξ		b	Causticum
4	B	Θ		c	Dulcamara
4	B	Γ		c	Pulsatilla
4	B	Σ		c	Sulphur

341

4	B	Z	d	Aurum met
4	B	Ψ	b	Ruta
4	C	H	c	Ignatia
4	C	Γ	b	Glonoine
4	C	Ω	e	Hepar sulph.
4	D	Ω	b	Aconitum.
4	D	Δ	b	Conium
4	D	Γ	d	Apis
4	A	Θ	b	Calcarea
4	A	θ	e	Kali carb.

INDEX